low carb
1 - 2 - 3

225 SIMPLY GREAT *3-INGREDIENT* RECIPES

low carb

1 - 2 - 3

ROZANNE GOLD

WITH HELEN KIMMEL, M.S., R.D.

RODALE

Printed in the United States of America
Rodale Inc. makes every effort to use acid-free ∞, recycled paper ♺.

Book design by Joanna Williams

Library of Congress Cataloging-in-Publication Data

Gold, Rozanne, date.
    Low carb 1-2-3 : 225 simply great 3-ingredient recipes / Rozanne Gold, with Helen Kimmel.
        p.   cm.
    Includes index.
    ISBN-13 978–1–59486–165–9 paperback
    ISBN-10 1–59486–165–X paperback
    1. Quick and easy cookery.   2. Low-carbohydrate diet—Recipes.   I. Kimmel, Helen.
  II. Title.
  TX833.5.G6498   2005
  641.5'6383—dc22
                                             2004022355

Distributed to the trade by Holtzbrinck Publishers

2 4 6 8 10 9 7 5 3   paperback

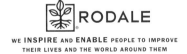

RODALE
WE **INSPIRE** AND **ENABLE** PEOPLE TO IMPROVE
THEIR LIVES AND THE WORLD AROUND THEM

FOR MORE OF OUR PRODUCTS
WWW.**RODALE**STORE.COM
(800) 848-4735

contents

preface

Our diet is like no other. Every recipe is low carb, low calorie, and low in saturated fat. Every recipe is based on fresh, natural ingredients. And every recipe uses only 3 ingredients!

Low Carb 1-2-3 was created not by laboratory workers in white coats, but by an award-winning chef working with a professional nutritionist to combine great cooking with optimal health. Our mission is to make it possible for you to eat more simply and healthfully every day. Here's how it works.

1-2-3 means:

- Recipes that use only three ingredients (except salt, pepper, and water)
- Recipes that are low not only in carbs but also in calories and saturated fat
- Recipes that are based on fresh, natural ingredients

Every recipe falls into one of three categories:

- VLC—very low carb (0 to 5 grams CTC)
- LC—low carb (6 to 10 grams CTC)
- ILC—indulgent low carb (11 to 18 grams CTC)

CTC, Carbs That Count, (total carbohydrates minus fiber) are listed for every recipe.

You can use these 1-2-3 recipes to:

- Lose weight
- Maintain your weight
- Eat a balanced, healthy diet

Here are more than 225 delicious recipes that are sure to simplify your life. *Low Carb 1-2-3* is designed to get you started—and to keep you going. Our special features make counting carbs easy as 1-2-3. Just add up the number of CTCs (and/or calories) to meet your daily—and lifelong—goals.

We say, "Three cheers for 1-2-3!"

Rozanne Gold and Helen Kimmel, M.S., R.D.
January 2005

acknowledgments

This book is dedicated to my magnificent mother, Marion Gold, and my late father, Bill (Bernard) Gold, whom I miss more than words can say. But since love grows exponentially, there is ample affection for my husband, Michael Whiteman, the smartest man in the world, who teaches me new things every day; and for my son, Jeremy Whiteman, who graciously gave up sugary drinks for awhile to help with our research. Whether my friends need to diet or not, I thank them for their warmth, wit, and wisdom, while I marvel at their accomplishments. They are worth their weight in carbs. Amy Berkowitz, Steve North, the incomparable Arthur Schwartz whom I cherish, Bob Harned, Dale Glasser Bellisfield, Phyllis and Ben Feder, Ann and Dan Feld (who inspired the idea for this book), Jonathan and Diana Rose, Rona Jaffe, Suzie Segal, Barry and MaryAnn Seidman, Diana Carulli, Erica Marcus, Robin Zucker and John East, Marcy Blum, Dr. Judy Nelson, Susy Davidson, Marc Summers, Barbara and Michael Cohen, Joanne and David Rosen, Audrey Appleby, Fern Berman, Laura Lehrman, Kate Merker, Tina Berry, Lila Gault, Ann Stewart, Lari Robling, Sally-Jo O'Brien, my "daughter" Anu Duggal (who understands the quotes), and Leon and Gail Gold, my very supportive brother and sister-in-law.

More thanks to my agent, Lydia Wills, who lights the way with her intellect and insight. Deep appreciation for my nutritionist and dear friend Helen Kimmel, who began the healthy journey with me more 15 years ago. Much gratitude to Barbara Fairchild and Kristine Kidd at *Bon Appétit* magazine. Professional thanks to everyone at Rodale, especially Miriam Backes, who has been so supportive and smart. Grazie mille to Rose Marie Morse for spreading the good news about the book in such a thoughtful and graceful way.

Most of all, thank you to all my readers who enabled the delicious spirit of simplicity to thrive.

—Rozanne Gold

This book is dedicated with love and respect to my parents, Brenda and Ed Rothstein. I try to live by their examples of kindness and compassion. They taught me that the most special times include our family and good friends—enhanced by great food and fine wine. Thank you for always believing in me!

To my husband, Barry, best friend and soul mate. Thanks for letting me follow my dreams and for eating all of my experiments. To my children, Robyn and Ian, who make my life complete, thanks for letting me have my "work time" so this book could become a reality. To Debra Bornstein, I'm so lucky to have you as my sister and friend.

To Rozanne Gold, my mentor and friend for more than 15 years, thank you for all the unbelievable opportunities and perfect advice you have given me. You truly are an inspiration!

To my fabulous New York girlfriends—Sabrina Laufer, Ilana Austin, Jodi Scheidlinger, Rhona Susser, and Jordana Barish—and to the "lovely ladies" of the South Jersey shore—Amy Hirsch, Emily Weiss, Jody Ludwig, Sandee Matlick, and Marva Nixon—it takes a village, and I'm glad you're in it!

To my in-laws, Rita and Morty Kimmel; my brothers and sisters-in-law, Brian Bornstein, Shari and Alex Salomon, Lauren and Steven Kimmel; and my Auntie Gail Bernstein, thanks for your encouragement.

Last, thanks to my grandmothers, Ida Rothstein and Helen Rothschild. Their memories and recipes fill my heart.

—Helen Kimmel

introduction

Everyone's doing it—eating low carb! But not the 1-2-3 way—not yet.

Low Carb 1-2-3 addresses the needs of everyone following today's profusion of low-carb diets. This uniquely versatile cookbook cross-references all the popular plans and establishes a common ground of recipes that work superbly for any low-carb program—including Atkins, the South Beach Diet, Sugar Busters, Glycemic Index diets, and many others.

Unlike other low-carb cookbooks, *Low Carb 1-2-3* is full of recipes that use only 3 ingredients. Herein lies the magic. As I have demonstrated in my award-winning 1-2-3 cookbook series, less truly is more. This innovative approach to keeping it simple unlocks the inherent flavors of the best ingredients, allowing them to shine through, unmasked and unmuddled.

And the 1-2-3 method goes one step further: Having developed hundreds upon hundreds of recipes in the course of my 25 years as a professional chef, I have discovered that *cooking simply also is the best way to eat healthfully.* When you have only three great ingredients in a recipe, there's little room left for the nutritional and gastronomic "bad stuff"—like excess sugar, white flour, saturated fats and trans fats, and overprocessed convenience foods. So this book's recipes are not only low in carbohydrates, but they are also low in calories and saturated fat. You will discover that a few fresh ingredients of uncompromising quality create remarkably satisfying results. And satisfaction is essential to anyone's success living a low-carb lifestyle.

I should know. I started my first diet at the age of 13. It was low-carb! (The craze actually began in the sixties.) And I lost 11 pounds in 2 weeks. I also tried low-cal diets and counting exchanges with my weight-watching parents for a while. Nothing lasted—except the vicious cycle from the euphoria of raiding the refrigerator when I was alone to the deep remorse and self-loathing that always followed. This near-anorexia and binging continued through college and into graduate school.

Then a funny thing happened on the way to size 16: I became a chef. It was a kamikaze career choice for someone who had been battling her weight since she was a teenager. But at the improbable age of 23, I became chef to New York Mayor Ed Koch, living and cooking at Gracie Mansion. The Mayor and I were *both* overweight, yet we devoured the homemade pasta I learned to make in Italy that summer, the dense cheesecake from Turf Bakery, New York bagels, and my famous chocolate mousse. We were carb crazy.

In my time off, I would hang out in the best kitchens of New York (Le Plaisir, Hoexter's, and La Colombe d'Or), working for free so I could hone my craft. I also ran my own catering business on the side. I had a love-hate relationship with food: loved to eat, hated my body. After Gracie Mansion, I became the youngest female executive chef in the country, developing menus for all of Lord & Taylor's department stores. Most of my crowd-pleasers were unhealthy: homemade cheese biscuits, buttery scones, flour-thickened creamed chicken in artery-clogging puff pastry shells, elaborate ice cream parfaits, and yes, of course, pasta. It was high-carb seduction.

Then I got the phone call that changed my life: Joe Baum, widely considered the greatest American restaurateur of the century, asked me to join his company. I became chef-director of the Joseph Baum & Michael Whiteman Co., the international restaurant consulting group best known for creating two of the world's most magical (and highest-grossing) restaurants—the Rainbow Room and Windows on the World (both the 1976 and 1996 incarnations)—as well as five of New York's finest three-star restaurants.

I always thought that I understood what people loved to eat. But now I was in for a big surprise: One of my responsibilities at Rainbow was to develop Evergreen, a healthy dining concept for members of the Rockefeller Center Club, who along with their checks got printouts detailing the nutritional value of the lunches they'd consumed. No longer able to seduce with carbs, I learned to deliver satisfaction by using a handful of superlative ingredients to create vivid, unadulterated flavors. The recipes combined ingenuity and optimal health. I started losing weight by eating my own food. And so did many guests, who were delighted with this new cuisine that broke all their misconceptions about what constituted healthy food. There was not a sprout in sight.

Helen Kimmel (then Rothstein)—the nutritionist for *Low Carb 1-2-3* and all my other 1-2-3 cookbooks—was instrumental in these innovations. I met her at the Rainbow Room in 1988. She was a registered dietitian with a master of science degree, and she helped me figure out the complex relationships between food and nutrition. Who knew?! We used olive oil and bits of butter and cream as top notes. All ingredients were always of the best quality. We dished up ample servings of protein. (Expecting anyone to feel satisfied with 3- or 4-ounce portions of meat, as do so many diets, is folly that guarantees failure!) We incorporated lots of fresh vegetables, fashioning faux fettuccine from asparagus peelings and angel hair "pasta" from slender strips of fresh zucchini. (I later came to recognize these as good carbs.) With Helen at my side, eagerly computing the amounts of bacon, cheese, and chocolate I could slip into a recipe, I created a new cuisine—one that applied French techniques and contemporary presentations to virtuous eating. *Cooking Light* magazine named me one of "America's Top 5 Enlightened Chefs."

Without knowing it at the time, we had created the ultimate low-carb, low-calorie diet.

And here it is. Recognizing how mightily people are struggling today at losing weight and then maintaining their weight loss—and having fought that battle myself—I have applied my simple formula to the lessons I have learned about healthy eating. Although *Healthy 1-2-3* (which won the prestigious IACP/Julia Child Award) is among the eight books in my 1-2-3 series, this is the first time I have created recipes specifically for those watching their carbs.

Perfect for today's hustle-bustle lifestyles, my 3-ingredient recipes make it easier to shop, to prepare, and to cook, too, because there are so few elements to deal with. 1-2-3 recipes make it possible to eat more simply and more healthfully every day.

the magic of 3 ingredients

Three is a powerful number in many disciplines—music, art, and poetry—so why not in cooking? I think of my recipes as flavor chords, in which unexpected flavors are combined in harmony and balance. The magic lies in employing clever techniques to coax forth intense, dramatic tastes. In cooking the 1-2-3 repertoire, only salt, pepper, and water—fundamentals to all cuisines—don't count as ingredients. Everything else does.

I often work 1-2-3 magic by exploiting an ingredient to its max. For example, in my recipe for Sautéed Turbot with Asparagus and Asparagus Velouté (page 177) steamed asparagus tips are served as a vegetable, atop the fish, and the stalks are boiled and whirled with a touch of sweet butter into a velvety sauce that finishes the dish. In Jade Zucchini Soup with Crab (page 76), crabmeat and zucchini are boiled and pureed, and then both ingredients are used as a garnish.

Clever application of simple techniques adds complexity to many dishes. In my Braised Hoisin Pork with Scallions (page 109), a robust shoulder of pork is first seared to maximize flavor, then slowly braised to reach ultimate tenderness. Turn to page 126 for an amazing recipe, in which a fillet of beef cooks in the oven for just 30 minutes, then sits on the kitchen counter bundled in newspaper until serving time, at which point it is perfectly cooked and still warm! And on page 108, white miso (a Japanese kitchen staple) transforms the flavor and texture of pork with delectably tender results.

And it's so easy! Working with just 3 ingredients dramatically reduces the effort and time spent prepping

healthy add-ons

Once you've mastered these recipes, you can augment them or garnish them with healthy add-ons that add flavor but no extra calories or carbs. These include grated citrus rind, chopped fresh herbs, a dusting of spice, a few celery leaves, a flourish of chive flowers, and hot pepper flakes. A teaspoon of fresh lemon juice or white vinegar adds only 2 calories and ½ gram of carbohydrates.

and cooking. Seeing a recipe come together from 3 simple components—or an entire meal from 12—is nothing short of fun.

something for everyone

Picture this: You're planning a dinner party, and you know that some of your guests are counting carbs, a few are concerned about fat intake, and a diabetic friend needs to eat low on the glycemic index. What to do? You can begin with a steaming bowl of Chardonnay Mussels (page 98) or a Baby Spinach Salad with Crispy Bacon (page 101) and follow with Chicken Rollatini with Salami and Roasted Peppers (page 142), Pesto-Crusted Rack of Lamb (page 113), or *Tournedos au Poivre* with Balsamic Syrup (page 121) as your main course. Add a side of some Simple Fried Cauliflower (page 199), serve fresh berries with Italian Zabaglione (page 254) for dessert, and . . . voila! You have a perfect low-carb, low-calorie meal that all of your guests can enjoy. As a friend of mine recently raved at one such dinner party, "It was the perfect balance of simplicity and seduction. Who knew healthy could taste like that?!"

With *Low Carb 1-2-3,* that is *exactly* what healthy tastes like. This cookbook makes it possible for everyone to enjoy the same meal without any sense of compromise, and it allows you, the host, to pull it off effortlessly.

Kids will love these recipes, too, especially the bright colors and appealing flavors and textures of such 1-2-3 finger food as Roast Beef "Kisses" with Chives (page 58) and Chicken-Pesto Satays (page 62), not to mention yummily healthy desserts like Strawberry and Toasted Almond Parfait (page 236). Imagine Smokey Joe Burgers (page 116), "Creamed" Spinach (page 214), and Chocolate-Tahini Cups (page 258) actually being good for you! Parents and kids can team up in the kitchen to make many of the recipes together and put a happy face on healthy eating.

low-carbing the 1-2-3 way

Because we care about your *health,* and not just weight loss, we care about more than just stream-lining carbs. So all of the recipes in this book are low in calories and saturated fat, too.

Because we know how important it is to eat good-for-you foods, we emphasize whole, fresh, un-processed ingredients; eliminate white flour and sugar; promote good fats of the poly- and mono-unsaturated varieties over saturated fats; eliminate artery-clogging trans fats altogether; and feature the good carbs—a lavish array of vegetables and fresh fruits that nourish the body and help main-tain health.

By giving you easy-to-follow, universally applicable guidelines, we empower you to follow any stage of any low-carb diet—whether it's Atkins, the South Beach Diet, Sugar Busters, or any other—with confidence. Simply determine your carb and/or calorie count for the day and choose recipes that add up to your goal.

While we've taken great pains not to overload you with data, we've included important nutritional information for each recipe: total carbohydrates and CTC (Carbs That Count), fiber, total fat and saturated fat, protein, and calories. So you can use this book even if you're not counting carbs, but just want to eat sensibly.

You may find this flexibility especially helpful after the initial phases of many low-carb plans, when you are left on your own to figure out how to maintain the diet.

To make it all easy, we offer some useful tools at the back of the book: 50 low-carb super snacks to satisfy every craving; 52 complete menus for breakfast, lunch, dinner, and special occasions; and a list of good-for-you foods that rate low on the glycemic index.

carb-counting made simple

Carb-counting can *seem* complicated, but our simple method makes it a snap. Carbs That Count (CTC) are listed for every recipe to differentiate between total carbohydrates and those that affect blood sugar levels. CTCs are calculated by subtracting the grams of fiber (which do not elevate blood sugar) from the total number of carbohydrates. It is these CTCs (also known as net carbs) that low-carb advocates are concerned about in determining daily carb intake.

To simplify carb-counting, every *Low Carb 1-2-3* recipe is marked with a symbol that tells you which of three categories it fits into:

■ VLC—very low carb (0 to 5 grams CTC)
■ LC—low carb (6 to 10 grams CTC)
■ ILC—indulgent low carb (11 to 18 grams CTC)

More than 58 percent of the recipes in this book fall into the very low-carb (VLC) category, 24 percent are low-carb (LC), and the remaining 18 percent are indulgent low-carb (ILC). This final category makes it possible to eat grains, fruits, and desserts.

So it's as simple as determining your target carb count for the day and choosing the recipes that add up to your goal. You can choose to have a 20-, 40- 80-, or even a 0-carb day! You can choose the recipes that sound most delicious to you, or you can look to the menu plans (page 268) for ideas.

Because I'm around food *all the time*—consulting for restaurants, creating recipes for my *Bon Appétit* magazine column "Entertaining Made Easy," and writing cookbooks—my weight sometimes moves upward unexpectedly. So I balance days of excess with days of restraint. But when I need to lose weight quickly and healthfully, I follow my own advice! For 2 weeks, I eat a varied menu—leaner proteins and low-glycemic vegetables and fruits—and hold to around 30 CTC a day, using the recipes in this book. Here's what a 1-2-3 day looks like when I'm aiming to lose weight:

Breakfast	CTC	Calories
Vermont Cheddar Frittata with Pickled Jalapeños (page 22)	2	197
Homemade Turkey Sausage (page 38)	1	102
French-press coffee	0	0
Lunch	**CTC**	**Calories**
Jade Zucchini Soup with Crab (page 76)	3	73
Halibut and Salmon "Osso Buco" (page 182)	.5	301
Poached Asparagus with Wasabi Butter (page 192)	3.5	117
Iced green tea	0	0
Dinner	**CTC**	**Calories**
Chilled Shrimp Cocktail with Low-Carb Cocktail Sauce (page 85)	6	129
Broiled Veal Steak with Fresh Thyme Mustard (page 129)	2	276
Sautéed Escarole with Garlic (page 201)	2	106
Strawberry Cheese Brûlée (page 237)	9	99
Glass of Chardonnay	1.5	120
Espresso	0	0
	Total CTC: 30.5	

For those counting calories, you may be surprised to know that the above plan adds up to just 1,520 calories! Not a bad diet, eh?

calories count, too

We've kept our recipes below 399 calories for main courses; under 199 calories for soups, vegetables, side dishes, and desserts; and under 275 calories for first courses and breakfasts.

We based our menus on an 1,800 calorie day, which can help you lose weight or maintain your weight. Much depends on your individual profile: your current weight, height, metabolism, and activity level. Simply choose the recipes that add up to your needs and desired caloric intake for the day. You will be amazed at the possibilities. For a sampling of low-carb menus that are also low calorie, turn to "52 Magical Menus" (page 268).

limiting saturated fat

Nutritionists worry that many low-carb diets oversell the idea that you can eat unlimited amounts of steak, bacon, butter, cream, and mayonnaise because they have almost no carbohydrates. And this is where most folks get into trouble. These foods are full of saturated fats and should be eaten in moderation.

We have restricted saturated fat to no more than 6 grams (rounded down) per recipe. Most have far less than that, and many rely on heart-healthy olive oil rather than animal fat. We trim visible fat from meat and remove the skin from poultry before eating. We use butter, bacon, and full-fat cheese in moderation to boost flavor and satisfaction, so there is no sense of deprivation. We have steered clear of *all* trans fats, the highly processed fats that can contribute to heart disease. Trans fats are found in a multitude of foods that line grocery shelves, particularly baked goods, crackers, and snacks.

sugar substitutes

Because sugar and honey are full of carbs and very high on the glycemic index, we have used sugar substitutes to keep our CTCs and calories low. We use sucralose (sold as Splenda), which is low-calorie, but *not* calorie-free, as many people think. While it does have less than 1 gram of carbs and 1 calorie per teaspoon, it adds up to 24 grams of carbs and 96 calories per cup. We believe that sucralose is the best-tasting low-cal sweetener, and we find that it stands up to heat in cooking better than other sugar substitutes. Also, it does not seem to affect insulin levels, which makes it a good option for diabetics. There are other low-calorie sweeteners on the market with taste you may prefer, but they don't work well in baking.

However, we do not advocate the use of sugar alcohol sweeteners such as sorbitol and maltitol because they are hard on the digestive system and their impact on insulin levels is now under question.

Here and there, we use limited amounts of a condiment or flavoring agent, such as hoisin sauce, that contains some simple sugars, but still fits our stringent criteria.

using 1-2-3 recipes with popular low-carb diets

We follow the guidelines set forth by the plans listed below as to which foods can be eaten freely, which should be limited, and which should be enjoyed only rarely (see "The *Low Carb 1-2-3* Food Lists" on pages 278 to 280). If you are in Phase 1 of the South Beach Diet or in the induction phase of Atkins, you should refer to your plan to see what the restrictions are for certain vegetables, fruits, and grains and choose 1-2-3 recipes accordingly. Remember that these severe limitations are temporary. After the first 2 weeks, you can freely use every recipe in this book as you continue into subsequent phases.

Use our CTCs as you do Atkins Net Carbs. For those just starting the ongoing weight loss phase of Atkins, your daily allowance of CTCs will be low, so focus on our VLC recipes. As you progress in your weight loss and move to weight maintenance, your daily CTCs can increase, so you'll have more flexibility to use our LC and ILC recipes.

what's the glycemic index?

The glycemic index (GI) ranks foods by their potential to rapidly increase blood sugar levels. This rise in blood sugar causes surges in insulin levels that have been linked to health problems, including high cholesterol and obesity. The GI originated as a tool for helping people with diabetes stabilize blood sugar.

Protein-rich foods such as poultry, beef, and fish all have very low GI numbers because they are very low in carbohydrates. Foods high on the index are refined sugar, white flour, and potatoes.

the south beach diet, sugar busters, and glycemic index–based diets

We have used whole, unprocessed foods that rank lower on the glycemic scale. *Low-Carb 1-2-3* adheres to the lists that the South Beach Diet, Sugar Busters, and Glycemic Index diets set forth detailing foods to eat freely and foods to limit. So if you're following any of these plans, you can use every recipe in this book with confidence once you've completed the strict induction phases.

about the nutritional data

Our nutritional analyses use the most up-to-date resources available, including two computer programs, USDA information, and many resource books.

For every recipe, we tell you the CTC, total carbohydrates, fiber, total fat, saturated fat, protein, and calories. We do not call for specific amounts of salt in our recipes, so if you are watching your sodium intake, you should determine how much is right for you. And unlike other cookbooks that obscure their nutritional information in microscopic typeface, or, worse, make health claims and don't give any nutritional information at all, we give it to you straight and gladly! These numbers will help you make simple decisions based on your personal needs.

start cooking!

Low Carb 1-2-3 cooking is easy, so you can basically jump right in. Here are a just a few pointers to help you achieve the best results.

- Read each recipe carefully and make sure you have all of the ingredients required.
- Whether you're a beginner or an expert cook, follow the instructions precisely. Be sure to use the right equipment and measure your ingredients.

- Don't make substitutions unless you've tried the dish first to understand its intention—the flavor, texture, and presentation.
- Keep in mind that altering a recipe could change its nutritional analysis. If you change one ingredient, you've changed one-third of the recipe!

If you're new to 1-2-3, you are going to be amazed by all the delicious things you can prepare with only three ingredients. It may change the way you cook and eat forever.

For those who have already discovered the pleasures of cooking à la 1-2-3, here's to your health!

the *low carb 1-2-3*
kitchen

Everyone wants recipes that work, but the outcome of cooking depends mightily on the ingredients you choose. Good ingredients are essential to simple cooking because when you cook with just three, there's nothing masking inferior quality.

So make a commitment to buy the freshest vegetables, herbs, and fruits—preferably in season—from a farmer's market or top-quality supermarket. A wise Japanese proverb states, "If you can capture the season on a plate, then you are the master."

And since all of these low-carb recipes are based on fresh, natural products, it's a good idea to make friends with your local butcher and fishmonger. Be willing to pay a little extra for the very best: hormone-free, free-range, organic, or products with pedigrees (Niman Ranch, D'Artagnan, Murray's Chickens, etc.). They tend to cost more, but they're well worth it. So are you.

the 1-2-3 pantry

Today, thankfully, there are many ingredients making up what I like to call a new world tapestry of flavors. You can impart new dimensions to familiar foods by making clever use of select items such as tandoori paste, light coconut milk, hoisin sauce, prepared pesto, even a good-quality jarred marinara sauce, plus staples like top-quality flavored olive oils and interesting vinegars (rice wine, balsamic, sherry, and raspberry). Also, there are a few—very few—"convenience" foods, such as chicken broth and jarred roasted peppers, that are indispensable in the 1-2-3 kitchen and appear in some of the recipes in this book.

About salt: Different kinds of salts vary in taste and in their effects on food. I generally prefer kosher salt for its bright taste and crystalline texture. I suggest you use it for most cooking and reserve coarse French sea salt for recipes that specifically suggest it.

About pepper: Please use freshly ground peppercorns for the best flavor. I have two pepper mills near my stove: a large one filled with black peppercorns and a smaller one filled with white peppercorns. Both black and white peppercorns are the small dried fruit of an East Indian plant. Black peppercorns are the unripe, sun-dried whole berry. White peppercorns are allowed to ripen completely and are the internal part of the berry; they taste remarkably different from black peppercorns, with a more camphor-like aroma.

Here's what else is in my pantry.

herbs, spices, and spice mixtures

Spices I use frequently are bay leaves, cumin seeds, fennel seeds, ground cumin, ground cinnamon, and star anise. All of my herbs, such as basil and parsley, are fresh.

The following spice mixtures can be found in specialty food stores and many supermarkets and are available by mail order from many specialty food sources.

- Za'atar: This intoxicating spice mixture from the Middle East (used in Lebanon, Jordan, Syria, and Israel), is made from dried hyssop, sumac, sesame seeds, and salt. It's available in Middle Eastern and spice markets.
- Five-spice powder: A staple of the Chinese kitchen made from cinnamon, anise, cloves, Szechuan peppercorns, and fennel, this is available in most supermarkets in the Asian section.
- Herbes de Provence: A combination of thyme, rosemary, lavender, savory, and sage, this is available in gourmet food stores, spice markets, and some supermarkets.
- Pumpkin pie spice: Made from cinnamon, ginger, nutmeg, and allspice, pumpkin pie spice is available in supermarkets.
- Smoked paprika: This is imported from Spain. The brand I use is La Chinata, and it is sold in small tins. It has a sweet, smokey fragrance and flavor. It's available in specialty/gourmet food stores.

convenience foods

All of the following ingredients can be found in good supermarkets.

- Chicken broth and beef broth: Choose low sodium, organic, if possible.
- Pesto sauce: Buy a good-quality jarred or refrigerated product.
- Marinara sauce: Look for one with fewer than 5 carbohydrates per ½ cup.
- Salsa verde: This is green, as the name implies, because it's made from tomatillos rather than tomatoes.

condiments

Most of these are available in good supermarkets; likely exceptions are noted.

- Olive oils: I use a good brand (such as Bertolli or Monini) of regular olive oil from the supermarket for almost all of my cooking. For recipes in which the flavor of the olive oil is especially important, I use extra-virgin olive oil—but not a very expensive one. I reserve my high-end extra-virgin olive oil for drizzling on salads.
- Flavored olive oils: These oils are infused with a variety of essences: Garlic and roasted garlic olive oils can be used interchangeably. (Roasted garlic has a more pronounced flavor.) Lemon, basil, and rosemary olive oils should be used as specified in each recipe. Buy a good brand such as Consorzio. "O" from California is an exceptional lemon olive oil. Good flavored oils are also imported from Italy. You may need to venture to a health food store or gourmet food market to find flavored olive oils, although they can be found in many supermarkets.
- Dark Asian sesame oil: This can typically be found in the Asian section of the supermarket.
- Roasted peanut oil: If it's not available at your supermarket, this oil can be found at health food stores.
- White truffle oil: Olive oil flavored with the essence of white truffles is sold in small bottles at specialty food stores.
- Vinegars: Red wine, balsamic, white balsamic, apple cider, raspberry, and sherry vinegars are all available at supermarkets; rice vinegar is often placed in the Asian section.
- Roasted peppers: Buy the jarred variety.
- Pickled jalapeños: Sold in jars.
- Sun-dried tomatoes in olive oil
- Light mayonnaise
- Dijon mustard
- Prepared white horseradish (not horseradish sauce)

reading labels

We encourage you to be a "food detective" because many similar products made by different companies have vast differences in nutritional values. Although we use a minimum of prepared food products, it is important to learn to compare nutrition labels and pick the product that's best for you. For example, when choosing pesto sauce, we recommend that you to select the one with the least fat and preservatives. When choosing a prepared marinara sauce, choose one with less than 5 grams of carbohydrates per ½ cup and make sure that sugar or any other sweetener is not one of the first five ingredients on the label.

It's especially important to always avoid products containing trans fats.

I also keep many "global" items on hand. These jarred or canned products are stocked in the ethnic section of many supermarkets. If your local grocery store doesn't carry them, seek out the specialty markets, health food stores, and ethnic food shops in your area. These items are well worth the trouble.

- Asian: Asian fish sauce, chili paste with garlic, hoisin sauce, light coconut milk, mirin (rice wine), teriyaki sauce, and wasabi powder
- European: black olive tapenade (generally imported from France, this spread comes in small jars)
- Indian: tandoori paste
- Indian/Southeast Asian: red curry paste
- Mexican: chipotle chile peppers in adobo sauce
- Middle Eastern: tahini (sesame seed paste, the best is available in jars in Middle Eastern markets and health food stores)

dessert ingredients

I keep these ingredients on hand especially for desserts.

- Granulated sugar substitute (Splenda or Equal)
- Light whipped topping (refrigerated)
- Sugar-free maple-flavored syrup (made with Splenda)

essential 1-2-3 refrigerator items

I make it a habit to keep my fridge stocked with these key ingredients.

- Extra-large organic eggs
- Unsalted butter
- Nitrite-free bacon
- Pancetta (thickly sliced)
- Smoked salmon (good quality)
- Low-fat, sharp Cheddar cheese
- Other cheeses (various; see individual recipes)
- Low-fat cottage cheese
- Neufchâtel cheese (instead of cream cheese)
- Plain, low-fat yogurt
- 1% milk
- Heavy cream
- Lemons and limes
- Fresh herbs (various)
- Onions
- Garlic
- Ginger (the fresh root)
- Champagne!

equipment 1-2-3

Every recipe in this book has been carefully analyzed, so it's important to measure your ingredients to ensure the exact carbohydrate and calorie amounts and other nutritional specifications. In order to do this, buy a small kitchen scale from a store that specializes in cooking equipment. They are inexpensive and fun to use. Also have two sets of measuring cups and measuring spoons. (I suggest two because I misplace mine all the time.)

Other than that, I live in a simple kitchen with no dishwasher, no microwave, and a minimum of pots and pans. What I find indispensable however, are a food processor and a hand-held mixer or a standing mixer with a large bowl. I have a blender for certain soups and sauce making, but in most cases, a food processor gets the job done.

Kitchen life would be unthinkable without my well-worn garlic press, a corkscrew, a microplane for grating citrus peel, a box grater for grating cheese and fresh ginger, a colander and a fine-mesh sieve, slotted spoons, ladles, and flexible rubber spatulas. Also essential are mixing bowls in a full range of sizes.

The pans I use most frequently on the stove top are 8" and 10" nonstick skillets and my 10" and 12" nonstick sauté pans with covers. I also rely upon a few large enamel Le Creuset casseroles or baking dishes, a 4-quart medium pot with a cover, a shallow roasting pan, and several rimmed metal baking sheets.

But most essential is my husband, who often cooks for me.

morning food

Most of us, even when we think we're starting the day with a healthy morning meal, typically wind up choosing between menus that are either high in carbohydrates or very high in saturated fat.

For example, a glass of orange juice, a bowl of cereal with milk and sliced bananas, and a cup of coffee with a teaspoon of sugar can add up to a whopping 91 CTCs! (96 carbs − 5 grams fiber = 91 CTC.) And it's easy to get in trouble with saturated fats: A three-egg cheese omelet with four slices of bacon may contain only negligible carbs, but it's loaded with 21 grams of saturated fat.

Meanwhile, those who think that eating light means stopping off at Starbucks to grab a toasted bagel with a smear of cream cheese and a "skinny" latte need a reality check, too. A 5-ounce bagel with 2 tablespoons of cream cheese and a latte made with ¾ cup skim milk add up to 82 CTC and 575 calories!

The good news is that you can enjoy rich and satisfying breakfasts that are low in carbs and saturated fats. This chapter offers you more than 25 delicious options, from hearty meals like Eggs à la Salsa (page 21) and Ham 'n' Eggs with Red-Eye Gravy (page 24) to lighter fare like Puffed Wheat with Blueberries and Milk (page 36) or Cantaloupe with Cottage Cheese and Mint (page 36). On page 26, you'll find "quick-quick" offerings for hectic workday mornings—in the time it

egg essentials

Eggs are central to a healthy low-carb diet, and they're incredibly versatile. Always keep a dozen in your refrigerator; they come in handy in myriad ways, any time of day. Italian-Style Fried Eggs (page 30) takes just 5 minutes to prepare and makes as delectable a lunch as it does a breakfast; a bowl of Chinese Marbled Eggs (page 27) is great to have on hand to snack on during the day, and Baked Eggs "Ranchero" (page 25) makes spontaneous Sunday brunch a snap.

A word of advice: Be gentle. Overcooking is eggs' worst enemy. Too much heat tends to alter their flavor and make them rubbery; this is true even of hard-boiled eggs. The obvious exception is Chinese Marbled Eggs, which requires 2 hours of simmering for the tea leaves and star anise to marble the eggs with color and infuse them with flavor. As a rule, I use extra-large eggs in the recipes, except where noted.

used to take to toast two slices of bread, you can whip up a fortifying breakfast such as Poached Eggs, Smoked Salmon, and Chives (page 26).

This chapter contains some wonderful surprises, such as crisp and subtly sweet Five-Spice Bacon (page 37) and addictive Homemade Turkey Sausage (page 38). Marvel at palate-pleasing Creamy, Lemony Eggs (page 28) that taste like real hollandaise sauce. Discover delightfully unexpected flavor combinations like Vermont Cheddar Frittata with Pickled Jalapeños (page 22) and the sophisticated pairing of Stir-Fried Eggs with Shiitake Mushrooms spiked with a little roasted sesame oil (page 35).

And there are luxuriant breakfasts for extra-special guests, or just treating yourself: delicious Frittata with Pancetta and Basil (page 23) or Eggs and Canadian Bacon, My Way, drizzled with a little white truffle oil (page 33).

Have a great breakfast and a great day!

breakfast quaffs 1-2-3

Fruit juices are notoriously high in carbohydrates. The following drinks satisfy the desire for something fruity and refreshing and still fit into one of our good-carb categories. Caloric content is low, too. Drink up!

morning lemonade

low carb	carbs that count
LC	9.5 grams

5   tablespoons freshly squeezed lemon juice (about 2 lemons)
2   tablespoons granulated sugar substitute
2   sprigs fresh mint

In a large glass, combine juice, sugar substitute, and ⅔ cup water and stir until the sugar substitute is dissolved. Stir in mint. Serve over ice with a thin slice of lemon.

Serves 1

CTC	9.39	Sat Fat	0
Total Carbs	9.82	Protein	.35
Fiber	.43	Calories	32
Total Fat	.02		

cranberry-lime juice

indulgent low carb	carbs that count
ILC	13 grams

2   tablespoons granulated sugar substitute
⅔   cup unsweetened cranberry juice
½   tablespoon freshly squeezed lime juice (about ½ lime)

In a large glass, stir the sugar substitute into ¼ cup water until dissolved. Add the cranberry juice and stir. Add the lime juice. Stir well and chill or serve over ice with a thin slice of lime.

Serves 1

CTC	12.90	Sat Fat	0
Total Carbs	12.9	Protein	.69
Fiber	.03	Calories	54
Total Fat	.01		

breakfast cider

indulgent low carb	carbs that count
ILC	17 grams

½   cup apple cider
1   tablespoon freshly squeezed lemon juice
1   tablespoon granulated sugar substitute

In a glass tumbler, combine the cider and lemon juice. In another glass, dissolve the sugar substitute in ½ cup water and stir into the cider. Chill well or serve over ice.

Serves 1

nutritionist's note: Fruit juice is a low-carber's forgotten pleasure. An occasional splurge is fine. In this refreshing cider, the glycemic load is lowered by the acidic lemon juice.

CTC	16.76	Sat Fat	0
Total Carbs	16.82	Protein	.06
Fiber	.06	Calories	70
Total Fat	0		

mango frullato

indulgent low carb	carbs that count
ILC	18 grams

2   tablespoons + 1 teaspoon granulated sugar substitute
1   very ripe medium mango, chilled
½   cup 1% milk

In a blender, dissolve the sugar substitute in ¼ cup water. Peel the mango and cut the flesh into 1" pieces. Add the mango, milk, a pinch of salt, and 6 ice cubes to the blender. Blend on high speed until thick and smooth. Serve immediately in chilled wine glasses.

Serves 2

CTC	18.04	Sat Fat	.46
Total Carbs	19.62	Protein	2.46
Fiber	1.58	Calories	90
Total Fat	.88		

mockachino

This has no coffee or caffeine, yet it tastes vaguely like a white chocolate cappuccino. Whisking the milk with a wire whisk during heating makes it incredibly frothy; it will fill a big mug and bring a big smile.

¾	cup 1% milk
1½	tablespoons sugar-free maple-flavored syrup
	Ground cinnamon

In a small saucepan, combine the milk and maple-flavored syrup. Begin to whip with a wire whisk and cook over medium-high heat until the milk is hot and the mixture is thick and frothy, about 3 minutes. Transfer to a warm mug and sprinkle with cinnamon. Serve immediately.

Serves 1

CTC	Total Carbs	Fiber	Total Fat	Sat Fat	Protein	Calories
10.27	10.71	.44	1.96	1.21	6.04	82

eggs à la salsa

You can buy shredded Monterey Jack cheese for extra ease in the morning or grate your own. This is quick, easy, and delicious.

2	extra-large eggs + 2 egg whites
¾	cup mild salsa
1½	ounces (about ⅓ cup) shredded Monterey Jack cheese

In a small bowl, whisk together the eggs and egg whites until thoroughly blended.

Coat a nonstick 9" skillet with cooking spray. Add the salsa to the skillet and cook over medium-high heat, stirring with a wooden spoon or flexible rubber spatula, just until hot. Add the eggs to the skillet and, using a flexible rubber spatula, fold the eggs into the salsa. Continue to stir while spreading the mixture into a thin pancake. Reduce the heat to medium and cook until the eggs are just set, about 2 to 3 minutes.

Scatter all but 2 tablespoons of the cheese on top of the eggs in the skillet. Cover the skillet and cook until the cheese is melted, about 1 minute longer. Remove from the heat. Cut the egg "pancake" in half using a spatula, then remove the eggs to warm large plates. Sprinkle each half with the remaining cheese and serve immediately.

Serves 2

nutritionist's note: We found that in this dish, a small amount of high-fat cheese works best yet still keeps CTC and sat fat within our limits.

CTC	Total Carbs	Fiber	Total Fat	Sat Fat	Protein	Calories
5.23	5.50	.27	11.71	5.60	16.05	195

vermont cheddar frittata with pickled jalapeños

This recipe's extra-long whipping time incorporates the peppers' pickling juice to create a texture that is light and custardy. You'll want to use a good Vermont low-fat cheddar for the best results.

½   cup sliced jarred pickled jalapeño chile peppers, reserving 2 tablespoons liquid

8   ounces (about 2 cups) low-fat shredded sharp cheddar cheese

10   extra-large eggs + 2 egg whites

Preheat the oven to 350°F.

With a paper towel, pat the chile pepper slices dry. Spray a 10" springform pan with a removable bottom with cooking spray. (If you don't have a springform pan, you can use a 12" nonstick skillet with an ovenproof handle.) Scatter the chile peppers evenly on the bottom of the pan. Sprinkle evenly with the cheese.

In a mixing bowl, combine the eggs and egg whites, ½ teaspoon salt, and a pinch of white pepper. Beat with an electric mixer on medium-high speed until very light, about 4 minutes. Add the 2 tablespoons reserved jalapeño liquid and mix briefly.

Pour the eggs over the cheese in the pan. Place the pan on a rimmed baking sheet and bake until just set and golden on top, 20 to 25 minutes. Remove the pan from the oven and let cool for at least 5 minutes before serving. (Frittatas generally taste better after they've rested.) Release from the springform pan. (If using a skillet, loosen the eggs with a plastic spatula.) Cut the frittata into wedges. Serve hot or at room temperature.

Serves 6

CTC	Total Carbs	Fiber	Total Fat	Sat Fat	Protein	Calories
2.03	2.26	.23	11.08	4.23	20.86	197

frittata with pancetta and basil

Frittata recipes in older cookbooks instruct you either to flip the eggs in the pan (at the risk of making a big mess on the stove top) or to turn the eggs upside down onto a plate and then slide them back into the pan. My technique of briefly running the frittata under the broiler achieves the same result without the juggling. Cilantro, mint, tarragon, and parsley can all be substituted for the basil with great success.

1   bunch fresh basil
3   ounces pancetta, sliced ¼" thick
7   extra-large eggs + 3 egg whites

Set aside several small sprigs of basil for a garnish. Now make a chiffonade: Stack 6 or 7 large basil leaves at a time and roll them tightly like a cigar. Hold the roll firmly and slice across into ¹⁄₁₆" strips. Repeat until you have ⅓ packed cup.

Cut the pancetta into ¼" dice and transfer it to a 10" ovenproof nonstick skillet. Cook over low heat for 8 minutes, stirring occasionally, until the pancetta barely begins to get crisp and the fat is rendered. (Do not let the pancetta brown.)

Meanwhile, in a mixing bowl, combine the eggs, egg whites, 3 tablespoons cold water, ¼ teaspoon salt, and freshly ground black pepper. Beat well. Pour the egg mixture over the pancetta in the skillet. Add the basil chiffonade. Reduce the heat to low, stir briefly with a wooden spoon, then let the eggs cook slowly, without stirring, for 1 minute. Cover the pan and cook until almost firm, about 7 minutes. (The eggs will set into a pale yellow color. Do not allow them to harden.)

Meanwhile, preheat the broiler. Place the frittata under the broiler, about 6" from the heat. Broil the frittata until it is just firm and the eggs take on color, for 30 seconds to 1 minute. Let it cool for about 5 minutes, then cut it into wedges and garnish with the reserved sprigs of basil.

Serves 4

nutritionist's note: Adding egg whites to whole eggs is a great way to increase the protein and portion size of this dish without adding any extra carbs or fat.

CTC	Total Carbs	Fiber	Total Fat	Sat Fat	Protein	Calories
1.51	1.77	.26	17.66	5.68	19.45	248

ham 'n' eggs with red-eye gravy

This is a classic 3-ingredient recipe that you might not expect to find in a "healthy" cookbook, but it fits into our lowest carb—and low saturated fat—category with ease.

2	large ham steaks (about 9 ounces each), with bone
½	cup freshly brewed black coffee
4	extra-large eggs

Trim the fat from the ham steaks and reserve it. Make several small incisions around the edges of each steak to help prevent curling. Cut the ham fat into small dice and set aside.

Heat 2 large nonstick skillets over medium-high heat until hot. Place 1 ham steak in each hot skillet and brown well, about 2 minutes on each side. Press down hard with a spatula to keep the ham from curling. Remove the ham to a warm platter and cut each steak in half.

Increase the heat under the skillets to high. Add ¼ cup of the coffee and freshly ground black pepper to each skillet and cook, scraping up the browned bits, until the sauce reduces slightly, about 1 minute. Pour the sauce over the ham. Cover the steaks with foil to keep them warm.

Carefully wipe out one of the skillets with a paper towel, set the skillet over high heat, add the ham fat, and heat until melted. Add the eggs to the skillet and quickly fry them to the desired firmness. Serve 1 egg atop each piece of ham. (This dish is best when the yolks are a bit soft so they run over the ham.) Add freshly ground black pepper to taste.

Serves 4

CTC	Total Carbs	Fiber	Total Fat	Sat Fat	Protein	Calories
.61	.61	0	9.83	3.18	28.42	213

baked eggs "ranchero"

I call this dish "ranchero" because of the tomato-cilantro combination, but you can substitute fresh basil, mint, or tarragon and call it what you wish.

2   cups V8 juice
1   large bunch fresh cilantro
4   extra-large eggs

Pour the V8 juice into a 10" nonstick skillet and bring to a boil. Reduce the heat to medium and simmer until the juice is reduced to 1 cup, about 10 minutes.

Meanwhile, set aside 4 sprigs of the cilantro for a garnish. Pluck the remaining leaves of cilantro and chop them roughly to yield ⅓ cup.

Raise the heat to high and bring the reduced juice to a boil again. Sprinkle the chopped cilantro over the juice. Carefully break the eggs over the cilantro into the sauce and reduce the heat to medium. Cook until the egg whites just begin to set, about 2 minutes. Cover the skillet and cook to the desired doneness. (I like to leave the yolks a little runny.) Garnish with the reserved cilantro sprigs and serve immediately.

Serves 2

CTC	Total Carbs	Fiber	Total Fat	Sat Fat	Protein	Calories
10.52	11.85	1.33	10.10	3.11	13.79	202

quick-quick breakfasts (ready in 8 minutes or less)

pita with cottage cheese and cucumber

low carb	carbs that count
LC	9 grams

½ cup 1% low-fat cottage cheese
¼ whole wheat pita (6" diameter)
¼ cup sliced cucumber

Spoon the cottage cheese onto a plate. Toast the pita and add it to the plate along with the cucumber slices. Sprinkle with salt and coarsely ground black pepper and serve.

Serves 1

CTC	9.08	Sat Fat	.74
Total Carbs	10.54	Protein	15.68
Fiber	1.46	Calories	120
Total Fat	1.56		

soft-cooked egg, bacon, and cottage cheese

low carb	carbs that count
LC	6.5 grams

1 extra-large egg
2 slices bacon
¾ cup 1% low-fat cottage cheese

In a small saucepan, place the egg with enough water to cover. Bring the water to a boil and boil until the egg is soft to medium-hard, about 3 minutes. (I prefer it soft-cooked.)

Meanwhile, in a skillet over medium heat, cook the bacon until crisp. Peel the egg and serve with the cottage cheese and bacon.

Serves 1

CTC	6.68	Sat Fat	4.51
Total Carbs	6.68	Protein	31.10
Fiber	0	Calories	267
Total Fat	12.75		

cottage cheese with cinnamon "sugar"

low carb	carbs that count
LC	6 grams

½ tablespoon granulated sugar substitute
½ teaspoon ground cinnamon
¾ cup 1% low-fat cottage cheese

In a bowl, combine the sugar substitute and cinnamon, sprinkle it on top of the cottage cheese, and serve.

Serves 1

CTC	5.91	Sat Fat	1.10
Total Carbs	6.53	Protein	21.05
Fiber	.62	Calories	125
Total Fat	1.77		

smoked salmon with whole wheat toast and "creamed cheese"

low carb	carbs that count
LC	7.5 grams

¼ cup 1% low-fat cottage cheese
¼ whole wheat pita (6" diameter)
3 ounces smoked salmon

In a food processor, blend the cottage cheese until creamy. Season with salt and freshly ground black pepper to taste. Toast the pita.

Arrange the salmon, pita, and cottage cheese on a plate and serve.

Serves 1

CTC	7.50	Sat Fat	2.25
Total Carbs	8.75	Protein	26.50
Fiber	1.25	Calories	195
Total Fat	6.88		

poached egg, smoked salmon, and chives

very low carb	carbs that count
VLC	.5 grams

1 extra-large egg
3 ounces smoked salmon
1 tablespoon minced fresh chives

Fill a small nonstick sauté pan with 1½" of water. Add enough salt so you can taste it and bring the water to a boil. Reduce the heat to medium. Crack the egg and carefully slip it into the simmering water. Poach the egg to desired doneness, about 3 to 5 minutes. Remove the egg with a slotted spoon and let it sit briefly on paper towels to drain.

Arrange the salmon on a plate. Set the poached egg next to or on top of the smoked salmon. Sprinkle all with coarsely ground black pepper, top with the chives, and serve.

Serves 1

CTC	.61	Sat Fat	3.55
Total Carbs	.61	Protein	24.24
Fiber	0	Calories	195
Total Fat	11.01		

chinese marbled eggs

Also known as "thousand-year-old eggs," a bowl of these marbleized eggs makes a fun, unexpected, morning meal. It is a rare preparation in which you purposely crack the shells. When you're ready to eat one, try sprinkling the eggs with a mixture of finely ground star anise, freshly ground black pepper, and salt.

12   extra-large eggs
6   tablespoons Darjeeling tea leaves
6   whole star anise

Place the eggs in a large saucepan with enough water to cover. Bring the water to a boil, then reduce the heat to a simmer and cook until the eggs are hard-cooked, about 10 minutes.

Using a slotted spoon, remove the eggs from the saucepan, reserving the water in the saucepan. Briefly run the eggs under cold water to cool. Add the tea leaves, star anise, and 1 tablespoon salt to the hot water in the saucepan and stir to combine.

Tap each egg lightly on a flat surface to make a web of small cracks all over the shell. Return the eggs to the saucepan, adding more water if necessary to cover the eggs. Bring the water to a boil. Reduce the heat and simmer, with the cover askew, for about 2 hours. Add more water if necessary to keep eggs covered. Let the eggs cool in the liquid, then transfer them to a bowl and refrigerate them until ready to serve. Store the eggs for up to 3 days. Peel the eggs before serving.

Serves 6

nutritionist's note: Keep a bowl of these eggs in the fridge for days when there's no time to prepare a low-carb breakfast—just grab and go. You can eat 1 whole egg and the whites of 2 more if you're watching your saturated fat intake.

CTC	Total Carbs	Fiber	Total Fat	Sat Fat	Protein	Calories
1.22	1.22	0	10.02	3.10	12.49	149

creamy, lemony eggs

These ultra-creamy eggs have the flavor of hollandaise sauce without all the saturated fat. Similarly, they are made in the top of a double boiler. This method is known as French-style scrambled eggs, and it is one of my favorite morning dishes.

6   extra-large eggs + 3 egg whites
1   lemon
2   tablespoons unsalted butter

In a mixing bowl, break the eggs and beat them thoroughly with a wire whisk. Add ¼ teaspoon salt and freshly ground black pepper. Grate the rind of the lemon to get 1 teaspoon zest and add it to the eggs. Cut the lemon in half and squeeze to get 2 teaspoons juice. Add the juice to the eggs and beat until mixed.

Place several inches of water in the bottom of a double boiler and heat until boiling. Reduce the heat to a simmer. Place the top of the double boiler over the water. Add 1 tablespoon of the butter and heat until melted.

Cut the remaining 1 tablespoon butter into tiny pieces. Pour the egg mixture into the top of the double boiler, then add the remaining butter. Cook, stirring constantly with a small rubber spatula or wooden spoon, until the eggs are thickened into soft curds, 10 to 12 minutes. Season with salt and freshly ground black pepper to taste and serve immediately.

Serves 4

CTC	Total Carbs	Fiber	Total Fat	Sat Fat	Protein	Calories
1.47	1.64	.17	13.28	5.91	12.10	177

breakfast tostada

Tostadas usually are made with tortillas that are fried crisp. I wanted to cut the fat, so I came up with this method, cooked under the broiler. Whole wheat pitas give you more fiber per square inch than the ordinary variety. This is a quick-and-easy recipe that your kids will especially like.

2   whole wheat pitas (6" diameter)
4   large plum tomatoes
4   ounces (about 1 cup) low-fat shredded cheddar cheese

Preheat the broiler.

Using a small, sharp knife, remove the outermost perimeter of each pita. Separate the pitas into 4 round halves. Place the pitas, inside side up, on a baking sheet.

Slice the tomatoes crosswise into paper-thin slices. Arrange tomato slices on each pita circle to cover it completely. Sprinkle the tomatoes with salt and freshly ground black pepper. Scatter the cheese evenly over the tomatoes. Set the baking sheet under the broiler, about 6" from the heat, and broil until the cheese is melted and bubbly. Serve immediately.

Serves 4

CTC	Total Carbs	Fiber	Total Fat	Sat Fat	Protein	Calories
15.93	19.79	3.86	3.14	1.29	10.96	145

fried eggs, italian-style

This simple recipe is adapted from one of my favorite cookbooks, The Flavor of Italy in Recipes and Pictures *by Narcisse and Narcissa Chamberlain, with black-and-white photos so evocative that they make you swoon. You could substitute a flavored olive oil such as basil or rosemary.*

2½ tablespoons extra-virgin olive oil
4   extra-large eggs
¼   cup freshly grated Parmesan or provolone cheese

Preheat the broiler.

Heat the oil in a medium-size ovenproof skillet over medium heat. Carefully break the eggs into the skillet and fry them until the whites are almost set, about 2 minutes. Remove the pan from the heat and sprinkle the eggs with a little salt, freshly ground black pepper, and the cheese. Set the pan under the broiler, about 6" from the heat, and cook until the cheese has melted, 3 or 4 minutes. Serve immediately.

Serves 4

CTC	Total Carbs	Fiber	Total Fat	Sat Fat	Protein	Calories
.80	.80	0	14.95	3.64	8.32	172

salami and eggs

You can use any salami for this dish, but tradition dictates Hebrew National, which is softer and more unctuous and garlicky than most other brands. Organic, preservative-free salami works great here, too!

2   ounces salami, thinly sliced
4   extra-large eggs
1   tablespoon finely minced fresh chives

In a medium nonstick skillet over high heat, cook the salami until it is lightly browned and some of the fat is rendered, about 2 minutes. Turn it over and cook 1 minute longer.

Into a medium bowl, break the eggs and, using a wire whisk, beat thoroughly with 1 tablespoon water and a pinch of salt and freshly ground black pepper. Pour the eggs over the salami and slowly cook, stirring with a wooden spoon or flexible rubber spatula until large soft curds form. Serve immediately, garnished with the chives.

Serves 2

CTC	Total Carbs	Fiber	Total Fat	Sat Fat	Protein	Calories
1.88	1.92	.04	15.73	5.40	16.49	220

open-face bacon-tomato pancake

This looks like a giant pancake, so I named it accordingly. It feeds two amply and is a satisfying way to start the day. Use nitrite-free bacon.

3   slices (about 1½ ounces) thick-sliced bacon
1   plum tomato, finely chopped
3   extra-large eggs + 2 egg whites

Cut the bacon into ½" pieces. In a medium nonstick skillet over high heat, cook the bacon for 2 minutes, stirring constantly, until it browns, gets a little crispy, and the fat is rendered. Add the tomato to the skillet and continue to cook over medium-high heat, stirring constantly, until the tomato softens, about 1 minute.

In a bowl, beat the eggs and egg whites until well blended. Add a very large pinch of salt.

Pat the bacon-tomato mixture into an even layer in the skillet. Pour the beaten eggs over the top. Cook over medium heat, loosening the edges of the eggs with a flexible rubber spatula, until the eggs are just set, about 3 minutes. Cover the skillet and cook until the tops of the eggs are just firm, about 2 minutes more. Carefully slide a spatula under the eggs to loosen the pancake. Turn out onto a warm large plate. Cut in half and serve immediately.

Serves 2

CTC	Total Carbs	Fiber	Total Fat	Sat Fat	Protein	Calories
2.36	2.70	.34	16.73	5.38	19.22	241

eggs and canadian bacon, my way

On the rare occasion that I cook only for myself, this is one of the dishes I make morning, noon, or night. It feels luxurious yet is surprisingly low in carbs and calories. A little truffle oil goes a very long way in supplying bold flavor. You can buy it at any gourmet food store and many supermarkets. Add a small salad and a glass of wine for a very stylish brunch.

¾   teaspoon white truffle oil
3   slices Canadian bacon
1   extra-large egg

In a medium nonstick skillet over medium-high heat, briefly heat ½ teaspoon of the oil. Add the Canadian bacon to the skillet and fry for 1 minute on each side.

Arrange the bacon in the skillet with the edges touching like a three-leaf clover, leaving a space in the center for the egg. Carefully break the egg into the center. Some of the white will spread across the bacon. Cook for 30 seconds and then cover the skillet. Cook until the egg white is firm and the yolk is still a little runny, 3 to 5 minutes. Using a spatula, immediately transfer the "pancake" to a warm large plate.

Drizzle with the remaining ¼ teaspoon oil and sprinkle with coarse salt and freshly ground black pepper. Serve immediately.

Serves 1

CTC	Total Carbs	Fiber	Total Fat	Sat Fat	Protein	Calories
1.50	1.55	0	14.27	3.99	23.15	235

poached eggs with buttered toast

Yes, it is possible to have eggs and buttered toast and still fit into a healthy eating plan.

4   extra-large eggs, chilled
2   slices whole wheat bread
2   teaspoons unsalted butter

Fill a 9" or 10" nonstick skillet with 1½" of water. Add enough salt so you can taste it and bring to a boil. Reduce the heat to a simmer and carefully break the eggs into the simmering water. Cook the eggs until just set, about 1 minute, then carefully loosen them from the bottom with a spatula. Continue to cook the eggs to the desired doneness, 3 to 5 minutes. Remove each egg with a slotted spoon and set it briefly on a paper towel to dry.

Meanwhile, toast the bread and spread it with the butter. Transfer the eggs to a warm plate and sprinkle with coarse salt. Cut each slice of bread in half on the diagonal and serve alongside the eggs. Serve immediately.

Serves 2

CTC	Total Carbs	Fiber	Total Fat	Sat Fat	Protein	Calories
12.30	14.15	1.85	15.06	5.75	15.26	252

stir-fried eggs with shiitake mushrooms

The beauty of this suave dish, in which exotic shiitake mushrooms provide an earthy Asian flavor and a texture that complements the eggs, is that it can be made for crowds. Its ingredients can easily be doubled as long as your wok is capacious enough.

5   ounces shiitake mushrooms

1   tablespoon roasted Asian sesame oil

7   extra-large eggs + 3 egg whites

Remove the stems from the mushrooms and discard. Wipe the mushrooms with a damp paper towel and slice them thickly on the bias.

In a wok over medium-high heat, briefly heat the oil. Add the mushrooms and cook, stirring constantly, until they begin to soften, 2 to 3 minutes. Add salt and freshly ground black pepper to taste and continue to cook, stirring, until the mushrooms are soft, about 1 minute longer.

In a bowl, beat the eggs and egg whites until thoroughly mixed. Add the eggs to the wok and cook over medium heat, stirring constantly with a flexible rubber spatula, scraping down eggs from the sides of the wok until they are scrambled to the desired consistency. (Be careful not to overcook; eggs are best when softly scrambled.) Serve immediately on warm plates.

Serves 4

CTC	Total Carbs	Fiber	Total Fat	Sat Fat	Protein	Calories
2.90	3.82	.92	12.41	3.22	14.40	185

cereal and fruit

puffed wheat with blueberries and milk

indulgent low carb	carbs that count
ILC	17 grams

½ cup blueberries
½ cup puffed wheat cereal
½ cup 1% milk

Wash berries under running water and dry well. Put the cereal in a bowl. Add the milk and top with the blueberries. Serve immediately.

Serves 1

nutritionist's note: High in powerful antioxidants, blueberries are a great addition to your carb-controlled morning.

CTC	17.17	Sat Fat	.85
Total Carbs	19.66	Protein	5.14
Fiber	2.49	Calories	111
Total Fat	1.79		

cantaloupe with cottage cheese and mint

indulgent low carb	carbs that count
ILC	14.5 grams

⅓ small ripe cantaloupe
½ cup 1% low-fat cottage cheese
1 tablespoon slivered fresh mint

Remove the seeds from the cantaloupe and transfer the cantaloupe to a plate. Place a mound of cottage cheese on top of the melon. Garnish it with the mint and serve.

Serves 1

CTC	14.3	Sat Fat	.84
Total Carbs	15.60	Protein	15.35
Fiber	1.30	Calories	134
Total Fat	1.58		

"sugared" strawberries with yogurt

indulgent low carb	carbs that count
ILC	16.5 grams

¾ cup sliced strawberries
3 teaspoons granulated sugar substitute
½ cup low-fat plain yogurt

Put the sliced strawberries in a bowl. Toss with 1 teaspoon of the sugar substitute and let them sit for 5 minutes.

In a small bowl, dissolve the remaining 2 teaspoons sugar substitute in 2 teaspoons water, then stir in the yogurt. Top the strawberries with the yogurt mixture and serve immediately.

Serves 1

CTC	16.38	Sat Fat	1.02
Total Carbs	19.24	Protein	6.76
Fiber	2.86	Calories	118
Total Fat	2.21		

grapefruit with cinnamon "sugar"

low carb	carbs that count
LC	9.5 grams

½ grapefruit
1 teaspoon granulated sugar substitute
¼ teaspoon ground cinnamon

Using a small knife or grapefruit knife, cut the grapefruit along the membranes to loosen the segments.

In a bowl, combine the sugar substitute and cinnamon and sprinkle on the grapefruit. Serve immediately.

Serves 1

CTC	9.58	Sat Fat	.02
Total Carbs	11.30	Protein	.83
Fiber	1.72	Calories	44
Total Fat	.15		

five-spice bacon

This is a great way to cook bacon. It gets crisp and doesn't shrivel as much as when you fry it in a skillet. Best of all, the smoky bacon gets a sugar-and-spice rub that makes it practically addictive. Five-spice powder, sold in most Asian markets and some supermarkets, is a Chinese mixture of cinnamon, anise, clove, Szechuan peppercorns, and fennel.

8   slices thick-sliced nitrite-free bacon (4 ounces)
2¼   teaspoons five-spice powder
1½   teaspoons granulated sugar substitute

Preheat the oven to 400°F.

Carefully separate the slices of bacon and place them on a rimmed baking sheet.

In a small bowl, mix together the five-spice powder, sugar substitute, and a large pinch of salt. Sprinkle the bacon with the spice mixture and rub it into the bacon to completely coat. Bake for 15 minutes, then pour off the fat. Bake for 5 to 10 minutes longer, or until crispy. Transfer the bacon to paper towels to drain. Serve hot.

Serves 4

CTC	Total Carbs	Fiber	Total Fat	Sat Fat	Protein	Calories
.99	1.69	.70	7.86	2.77	4.88	97

homemade turkey sausage

It is incredibly satisfying to make your own sausage, and you can do it in just 5 minutes. This version is made in patties and is so much better than anything you can buy in the supermarket. It is preservative-free with a vivid taste. It is also low calorie with very little saturated fat compared to most other sausages. You can use ground all-white turkey breast meat or the more standard ground turkey, which is a combination of light and dark meat. I've supplied the nutritional analysis for both.

12   ounces ground turkey
4   cloves garlic
2   teaspoons ground cumin

In a medium-large bowl, place the ground turkey. Press the garlic through a garlic press and add it to the turkey. Add the cumin, ½ teaspoon salt, and a heaping ¼ teaspoon freshly ground black pepper. Using a fork, mash the ingredients to incorporate them. Cover and refrigerate for up to 1 hour to let the flavors mingle, or you can cook it immediately.

Using your hands, form the mixture into 12 flat patties, each about 2" in diameter and about ¼" thick.

Heat a large nonstick skillet over medium-high heat until hot. Add the sausage patties and cook them on one side until browned, about 2 minutes. Carefully turn the patties over and cook them on the other side until browned and just cooked through, about 2 minutes longer. (Do not overcook; you want the patties to be moist.) Serve immediately.

Serves 4

nutritionist's note: By choosing this wonderful sausage over store-bought pork sausage, you save a whopping 23 grams of saturated fat for each serving.

all-white ground turkey

CTC	Total Carbs	Fiber	Total Fat	Sat Fat	Protein	Calories
.93	1.39	.46	.63	.14	20.96	102

light and dark ground turkey

CTC	Total Carbs	Fiber	Total Fat	Sat Fat	Protein	Calories
.93	1.39	.46	7.24	1.92	15.24	137

turkey sausage, poached egg, and broiled tomato

If you don't have time to make your own sausage, you can still have this delicious breakfast by purchasing a good-quality brand of turkey sausage. Choose the one with the least fat and preservatives.

2	turkey breakfast sausages (about 2½ ounces total)
1	plum tomato
1	extra-large egg

Preheat the broiler.

In an 8″ × 8″ baking dish, place the sausages. Cut the tomato in half through the stem end and sprinkle it lightly with salt and freshly ground black pepper. Add the tomato to the baking dish. Set the baking dish under the broiler, about 6″ from the heat, and broil for 5 to 7 minutes, until the sausages are cooked through and the tomato is slightly charred.

Fill a small skillet with 1½″ of water. Add enough salt so you can taste it and bring the water to a boil. Reduce the heat to medium. Crack the egg and carefully slip it into the simmering water. Poach the egg to the desired doneness, about 3 to 5 minutes. Remove the egg with a slotted spoon and let it sit briefly on paper towels to drain. Transfer the egg to a plate, sprinkle it lightly with salt, and serve with the sausages and tomato.

Serves 1

CTC	Total Carbs	Fiber	Total Fat	Sat Fat	Protein	Calories
3.31	3.99	.68	13.97	5.33	21.52	228

party food

Once upon a time, party food meant mega-carbs in every bite: canapés and toasts, puff pastry barquettes, asparagus baked in sheaths of butter-doused white bread, miniature pizzas, pigs-in-blankets, nachos, and stuffed potato skins!

Today's cocktail parties are witness to a new age of carb-conscious guests lifting the shrimp from the canapé, jettisoning the rice from the sushi, slurping the guacamole *off* the tortilla, and eating cheese *without* crackers. One would sooner plunge one's finger into the onion dip than use a potato chip.

Savvy and gracious party givers won't burden their guests with heavy, starchy hors d'oeuvres containing unwanted—or, worse, hidden—carbs. This chapter shows you just how easily and deliciously you can rise to this challenge.

Great low-carb hors d'oeuvres come in myriad forms—from classic crudités served with delectably low-carb dips (pages 43 to 47) to canapés that employ disks of cucumber or rounds of zucchini rather than slices of bread, such as Rosettes of Smoked Salmon (page 53) and Chicken-Pesto Satays (page 62) to Wasabi-Stuffed Shrimp (page 55). And don't hesitate to look outside this chapter for recipes that translate easily into hors d'oeuvres. Tiny cups of some soups (pages 69 to 82) qualify as party food, as do various items from the Morning Food chapter, including small squares of a frittata—Vermont Cheddar Frittata with Pickled Jalapeños (page 22) or Frittata with Pancetta and Basil (page 23)—and quarter-size Homemade Turkey Sausage patties flavored with cumin (page 38). A platter of Simple Fried Cauliflower (page 199) from the Vegetables and Side Dishes chapter makes a terrific low-carb finger food. And what finicky carbophobe wouldn't be delighted by Peppered Tuna "Tataki" (page 88) or Chilled Shrimp Cocktail with Low-Carb Cocktail Sauce (page 85), both of which are found in the Soups and Starters chapter? Included in *this* chapter are 24 quick and easy ideas—reason enough to celebrate.

Where there's food, there's often drink. Distilled spirits such as gin, vodka, rum, and bourbon are all carb-free—but this is not license to imbibe with abandon. Generally, wine is a healthier, less caloric choice (see "Low-Carb Wines and Beer" below). Sparkling wine—real champagne from France, Cava from Spain, and Prosecco from Italy—or a great domestic sparkler—such as Gruet (New Mexico), Schramsberg (California), or Clinton Vineyards (New York)—is the best way to jump-start any party. Be sure to choose one that is "brut" (extremely dry); it will have the least residual sugar and carbs. Cheers!

low-carb wines and beer

You will be delighted to know that wine, and even an occasional beer, can be part of a healthy low-carb diet. Wine, especially red wine, contains heart-healthy polyphenols, which are believed to reduce the risk of heart disease and some kinds of cancer. (Note: Certain low-carb programs suggest avoiding any alcohol during their initial phases.)

Hard spirits, such as vodka, scotch, rum, etc., while low in carbohydrates, are high in calories and have almost no nutritive value.

The following analysis for wine is based on dry white, rose, and red wines, with imperceptible amounts of residual sugar. Calculations are based on 5 glasses of wine per bottle. There are many low-carb beers on the market now, so check the labels.

white wine and dry sparkling wine, 5-ounce glass

CTC	1.18	Sat Fat	0
Total Carbs	1.18	Protein	.15
Fiber	0	Calories	100
Total Fat	0		

rose wine, 5-ounce glass

CTC	2.06	Sat Fat	0
Total Carbs	2.06	Protein	.30
Fiber	0	Calories	105
Total Fat	0		

red wine, 5-ounce glass

CTC	2.50	Sat Fat	0
Total Carbs	2.50	Protein	.29
Fiber	0	Calories	105
Total Fat	0		

dry sherry, 4-ounce glass

CTC	2.4	Sat Fat	0
Total Carbs	2.4	Protein	0
Fiber	0	Calories	126
Total Fat	0		

light beer, 12-ounce glass

CTC	4.50	Sat Fat	0
Total Carbs	4.50	Protein	.71
Fiber	0	Calories	99
Total Fat	0		

white wine spritzer

very low carb	carbs that count
VLC	1 gram

Instead of the lemon peel, sometimes I add a few drops of angostura bitters.

1   strip lemon peel
3½ ounces dry white wine, chilled
    Chilled seltzer, plain or
    flavored

Rub the lemon peel around the edge of a large wine glass. Add a few ice cubes to the glass and pour the wine over. Top with seltzer and drop in the lemon peel.

Serves 1

CTC	.83	Sat Fat	0
Total Carbs	.83	Protein	.11
Fiber	0	Calories	70
Total Fat	0		

roasted pepper dip

This dip will remind you of old-fashioned pimiento cheese. I've specified Neufchâtel, the low-fat version of cream cheese, because you don't need the extra calories and it works perfectly well with this party-colored dip.

8   ounces Neufchâtel (low-fat) cream cheese
½   cup jarred roasted peppers, drained
2   tablespoons finely minced fresh chives

Break up the cheese into several pieces and add to a food processor. Pat the peppers dry with paper towels, chop the peppers coarsely, and add them to the food processor. Process the mixture until very smooth, slowly adding 1 tablespoon cold water. Add salt and freshly ground black pepper to taste.

Transfer the mixture to a serving bowl. Stir in 1 tablespoon of the chives. Scatter the remaining chives on top. Cover and refrigerate until cold.

Serves 12 (2 tablespoons per serving)

nutritionist's note: Some light cream cheeses are made of Neufchâtel, and others are made from a combination of foods including high-carb food starch. Check the ingredient listings and buy the one that specifies Neufchâtel.

CTC	Total Carbs	Fiber	Total Fat	Sat Fat	Protein	Calories
.26	.27	.01	4.00	2.67	2.02	48

smokey eggplant-pesto dip

Roasting the eggplant until the skin blackens and chars creates a deliciously smokey aroma and flavor.

1	large eggplant (about 1½ pounds)
¼	cup prepared pesto
1	large lemon

Preheat the oven to 400°F.

Place the eggplant directly over the open fire of a stove-top burner or place it on a baking sheet under the broiler, about 6" from the heat. Cook for a few minutes, rotating the eggplant with tongs so that the skin blisters and chars all over.

Transfer the eggplant to a baking sheet (if it's not already on one) and bake for 50 minutes, turning once halfway through the cooking time. Remove from the oven. Cut the eggplant in half lengthwise and let it cool. When the eggplant is cool enough to handle, scoop out the flesh and transfer it to a food processor. Add the pesto. Grate the zest of the lemon and add it to the food processor. Halve the lemon and squeeze it to get 2 tablespoons juice. Add the juice to the food processor and process until the ingredients are incorporated and the mixture is fairly smooth. (Do not overprocess; you want the dip to have some texture.)

Transfer the dip to a serving bowl. Add salt and freshly ground black pepper to taste. Cover and refrigerate until cold.

Serves 12 (2 tablespoons per serving)

nutritionist's note: Remember to compare the nutrition labels on different brands of pesto. Choose the one with the least fat; I often find that the store brand is the best choice.

CTC	Total Carbs	Fiber	Total Fat	Sat Fat	Protein	Calories
1.86	3.13	1.27	.91	.21	.87	22

cucumber-chive dip

Since grated cucumber is watery, I use low-fat sour cream in this recipe. It maintains its texture better than yogurt would. This dip is great for dipping bell pepper strips into instead of taco chips.

¾   cup low-fat sour cream
½   cucumber
1   large bunch fresh chives

In a small bowl, place the sour cream. Peel the cucumber and grate it on the large holes of a box grater. Add the grated cucumber and its juices to the bowl. Finely mince the chives to get about ¼ cup. Stir the minced chives into the cucumber mixture. Add salt and freshly ground black pepper to taste. Cover and refrigerate until cold.

Serves 8 (2 tablespoons per serving)

CTC	Total Carbs	Fiber	Total Fat	Sat Fat	Protein	Calories
3.34	3.50	.16	1.54	.76	1.65	33

tahini dip with lime

For a change of pace, I prepare this tahini dip with fresh lime zest and juice instead of the more usual lemon. Tahini resembles peanut butter and is found in Middle Eastern markets, health food stores, and even many supermarkets. Use this as a dip for almost any raw vegetable or for nuggets of grilled fish such as tuna or swordfish. I love this dip with raw jícama, a sweet, crunchy, potato-like tuber found in most supermarkets. One cup of jícama slices is fat free and has only 4.7 grams CTC.

½   cup tahini (sesame seed paste)
2   limes
1   large clove garlic

Stir the tahini in the jar, making sure to incorporate any oil that may have risen to the top. Scoop out ½ cup and place it in a food processor. Grate the zest of 1 lime and add it to the processor. Halve the limes and squeeze ¼ cup juice. Add the juice to the processor. Add the garlic, pushed through a garlic press. Process the mixture while slowly adding ½ cup cold water until you have a smooth, thick puree.

Transfer the mixture to a serving bowl. Add salt and freshly ground black pepper to taste. Add more cool water, if needed. Chill until ready to serve.

Serves 8 (2 tablespoons per serving)

CTC	Total Carbs	Fiber	Total Fat	Sat Fat	Protein	Calories
3.32	4.75	1.43	7.21	1.01	2.73	88

roquefort-basil dip

Here, pungent Roquefort cheese is mellowed by cottage cheese, which also balances its higher fat content. The result is a flavorful low-carb, low-fat dip. This is especially delicious as a dip for grape tomatoes. I generally thread them on the tips of 6" bamboo skewers and let guests dip away!

1	large bunch fresh basil
2	cups 1% low-fat cottage cheese
4	ounces Roquefort cheese

Chop enough basil to yield ½ loosely packed cup.

In a food processor, place the cottage cheese. Crumble the Roquefort cheese and add it to the processor. Briefly process until just blended. Add the basil and process until very smooth. Season with salt and freshly ground black pepper. Chill before serving.

Serves 16 (2 tablespoons each)

CTC	Total Carbs	Fiber	Total Fat	Sat Fat	Protein	Calories
1.40	1.45	.05	2.43	1.62	4.56	47

smoked pecans

These nuts are always offered in my house; they seems to disappear magically from the nut bowl.

2   tablespoons unsalted butter
8   ounces (2 cups) large pecan halves
2   teaspoons smoked paprika (see "The 1-2-3 Pantry" on page 12)

Preheat the oven to 250°F.

In a large nonstick skillet over medium heat, melt the butter. Add the pecans, 1½ teaspoons of the paprika, 1 teaspoon salt, and a generous grinding of black pepper. Cook, stirring well, until the pecans are coated, about 1 minute.

Transfer the pecans to a parchment-lined baking sheet and bake for 20 to 25 minutes, stirring once. (Do not let the pecans get too dark, or they will taste bitter.) Toss them with a little more of the remaining smoked paprika, to taste. Remove the pecans from the oven, transfer them to paper towels to drain, and let them cool to room temperature before serving. Store in a tightly covered tin or jar.

Serves 16 (about 8 pecans per serving)

CTC	Total Carbs	Fiber	Total Fat	Sat Fat	Protein	Calories
.79	2.15	1.36	11.83	1.77	1.50	112

lemon almonds with dill

These are perky and fresh-tasting, with the dill providing a surprising overtone. You also can make this recipe with slivered almonds. Blanched almonds can be found in health food stores. You can also blanch your own by adding almonds with skins to boiling water to cook for 30 seconds; the skins will then slip off easily.

1   bunch fresh dill
¼   cup lemon oil (see "The 1-2-3 Pantry" on page 13)
10 ounces (2 cups) whole blanched almonds

Finely chop the dill and set it aside.

In a very large nonstick skillet over medium-high heat, heat the oil. Add the almonds and cook for 1 minute. Add ¼ cup of the chopped dill to the skillet and cook, stirring constantly, until the almonds are golden and the dill becomes crispy, 5 to 7 minutes. Add salt and freshly ground black pepper to taste. Transfer the almonds to paper towels to drain. Cool to room temperature before serving and garnish with more chopped dill. Store in a tightly covered tin or jar.

Serves 16 (about 15 almonds per serving)

CTC	Total Carbs	Fiber	Total Fat	Sat Fat	Protein	Calories
2.30	4.54	2.24	12.83	1.18	4.26	141

glazed walnuts

Walnuts have become the darling of the nut world. They are full of nutrients and purported to help circulation. You'll be surprised at the mysterious sweet taste contributed by the Worcestershire sauce.

2   tablespoons garlic oil
2   cups walnut halves
2½   tablespoons Worcestershire sauce

In a large nonstick skillet over medium-high heat, heat the oil. Add the walnuts and cook, stirring constantly, until the nuts are browned, about 3 minutes. (Be careful not to overcook.) Add the Worcestershire sauce and continue to cook, stirring, for 1 minute longer. Add a pinch of salt and freshly ground black pepper, stir, and remove from the heat.

Using a slotted spoon, transfer the nuts to a piece of parchment or waxed paper and let cool before serving. Store in a tightly covered tin or jar.

Serves 16 (about 6 nuts per person)

nutritionist's note: Walnuts are a great source of omega-3 fatty acids (the fat most commonly associated with fish), which can help lower triglycerides and raise your good HDL cholesterol.

CTC	Total Carbs	Fiber	Total Fat	Sat Fat	Protein	Calories
1.34	2.18	.84	10.31	.99	2.37	99

whole wheat pita chips

In the low-carb world, where most bread is forbidden, these chips are a blessing. You could substitute freshly grated Parmesan cheese, but I like the bite of pecorino.

2   whole wheat pitas (6" diameter)

3   tablespoons extra-virgin olive oil

⅓   cup freshly grated pecorino Romano cheese

Preheat the oven to 350°F.

Cut each pita into 8 equal-size pie-shaped wedges. Gently separate each wedge into 2 triangular pieces. (You will have 32 pieces.) Using a pastry brush, lightly brush each triangle with oil. Sprinkle each triangle with a little cheese.

Place the pita triangles on a rimmed metal baking sheet. Bake for 5 to 6 minutes, until just crisp. (Be careful not to overcook.) Remove the chips from the oven and cool to room temperature.

Serves 16 (2 chips per serving)

CTC	Total Carbs	Fiber	Total Fat	Sat Fat	Protein	Calories
2.82	3.44	.62	3.22	.66	1.44	48

anchovy-stuffed celery

For as long as I can remember, my mother served anchovy cream cheese at her cocktail parties. It is a great tidbit to accompany the occasional martini.

8   ounces Neufchâtel (low-fat) cream cheese
1   can (2 ounces) rolled anchovies with capers, drained
1   bunch celery

In a food processor, place the cream cheese. Add the anchovies and capers to the food processor. Process the mixture until smooth. Add salt, if needed, and freshly ground black pepper to taste. Chill until ready to use.

Remove the outer stalks from the celery and save for another use. Separate the remaining stalks, wash them well, and pat dry with paper towels. Mince some of the celery leaves to get ¼ cup and set aside. Cut the celery stalks into 32 1½" lengths. Using a small knife, fill the celery with the cheese mixture, mounding on top. Sprinkle with the chopped celery leaves and serve.

Serves 16 (2 per serving)

nutritionist's note: Neufchâtel can be found next to the cream cheese in your supermarket. Beware of imitations that use carb-laden food starch.

CTC	Total Carbs	Fiber	Total Fat	Sat Fat	Protein	Calories
.34	.64	.30	3.30	2.06	2.44	44

rosettes of smoked salmon

This is easy, elegant, and perfect for low-carb cocktail parties. These are nice with a glass of dry rose champagne.

4 small kirby cucumbers (about 1" in diameter)
½ pound very thinly sliced smoked salmon
⅓ cup whipped cream cheese

Trim ends from cucumbers and discard. Cut each cucumber into 6 uniform ¼"-thick slices. Pat dry with paper towels.

Slice the smoked salmon into 1"-wide by 3"-long strips to make 24 pieces. Roll each piece loosely. Curl back the edges of each piece and flatten slightly so that it begins to look like a rose.

Spread about ½ teaspoon cream cheese on each cucumber slice and place a salmon rosette on top. Fill the center of each rosette with ¼ teaspoon cream cheese. Arrange them on a platter and serve.

Serves 12 (2 rosettes per serving)

CTC	Total Carbs	Fiber	Total Fat	Sat Fat	Protein	Calories
.74	1.04	.30	2.94	1.46	4.48	47

smoked salmon "pâté" with pita crisps

I wanted to create a creamy nondairy party dish and so tried Tofutti spread, a soy-based cream cheese look-alike. Void of any flavor, tofutti turns out to be a great flavor-carrier. No one will know the difference, and you can serve it at a kosher meal! Crisp pita chips add a nice textural contrast. Choose a heavily smoked salmon for this recipe.

3   ounces smoked salmon

8   ounces Tofutti

2   whole wheat pitas (6" diameter)

Cut the salmon into large pieces and place it in a food processor with the Tofutti. Process until thoroughly blended. Add salt and freshly ground black pepper to taste and mix. Transfer to a bowl and refrigerate until cold.

Preheat the oven to 350°F.

Cut each pita into 8 wedges. Separate each pita wedge into 2 triangles. Place the pita triangles, inside side up, on a baking sheet. Bake for 5 to 6 minutes, until crisp. (Do not let them get too brown.) Remove them from the oven and let cool.

To serve, put a heaping teaspoon of smoked salmon "pâté" on each pita crisp and place it on a decorative plate.

Serves 16 (2 pieces per serving)

CTC	Total Carbs	Fiber	Total Fat	Sat Fat	Protein	Calories
3.24	3.87	.63	4.56	1.12	2.37	65

wasabi-stuffed shrimp

This has become a classic at my dinner parties, served with small glasses of chilled sake. To satisfy my low-carb and low-saturated-fat mandate, I've substituted Neufchâtel for regular cream cheese. If you're short on time, you can buy precooked shrimp.

32 jumbo shrimp in their shells (about 2 pounds)
8 ounces Neuchâtel (low-fat) cream cheese
2 tablespoons wasabi powder

Wash the shrimp under cold, running water. Bring a large pot of water to a boil. Add enough salt to make the water taste very salty. (This is the secret to making great shrimp!) Add the shrimp (still in their shells) to the pot, reduce the heat to medium, and cook until the shrimp are just firm, 3 to 4 minutes. Using a slotted spoon, transfer the shrimp to a bowl of ice cold, heavily salted water to cool. Drain well. Pat dry with paper towels and chill until ready to use.

In a food processor, place the cream cheese.

In a small bowl, mix the wasabi powder with 1½ to 2 tablespoons cold water to form a thick paste. Add the wasabi paste to the food processor with ¼ teaspoon salt or more to taste. Process until smooth. Chill until ready to fill the shrimp.

Peel and devein the shrimp. Using a small knife, split the shrimp down the back, cutting about two-thirds of the way through. Using a small spoon or pastry bag, stuff each shrimp with 1½ teaspoons wasabi cream cheese. Press the sides gently together and arrange the stuffed shrimp on a serving platter.

Serves 16 (2 shrimp per serving)

CTC	Total Carbs	Fiber	Total Fat	Sat Fat	Protein	Calories
.68	.76	.08	3.99	2.19	13.06	96

cherry tomatoes with herbed cheese

A cinch to make, herbed cheese is delicious as a dip for other raw vegetables, especially fresh fennel. I find it festive to serve these stuffed tomatoes in individual 1" fluted paper cups, the kind that's generally used for candy. They come in many colors and patterns and can be found in party stores.

½ cup farmer cheese
3 tablespoons prepared pesto
36 medium cherry tomatoes

Into a food processor, crumble the farmer cheese. Add the pesto and process until smooth and the ingredients are uniformly blended. (Do not overprocess.) Add salt and freshly ground black pepper to taste and mix. Transfer to a small bowl. (You will have about ¾ cup.) Cover and refrigerate until firm.

Cut a small slice from the top (stem end) of each tomato. Scoop out the pulp with a small spoon, leaving the tomato shells intact. Discard the pulp. Fill each tomato with chilled herbed cheese. Serve immediately or chill until ready to serve.

Serves 18 (2 tomatoes per serving)

CTC	Total Carbs	Fiber	Total Fat	Sat Fat	Protein	Calories
1.08	1.38	.30	1.06	.46	1.17	19

prosciutto-honeydew-mint brochettes

These sweet-salty brochettes also can be made with chunks of mango wrapped with air-dried beef known as bresaola. I just love the way these go with brut champagne. You'll need 40 4" bamboo skewers to serve these on.

1	small ripe honeydew
10	thin slices prosciutto (about ¼ pound)
1	bunch fresh mint

Cut the honeydew in half through the equator and discard the seeds. Using a large melon baller, scoop out 40 melon balls. Pat the melon balls dry with paper towels, and lightly sprinkle with freshly ground black pepper and a pinch of salt.

Cut the prosciutto in half across the width and then along the length to get 40 ribbon-shaped pieces. Wrap each melon ball with a piece of prosciutto.

Place 1 wrapped melon ball on each of 40 4" bamboo skewers. Place the skewers on a large serving plate.

Stack the largest mint leaves and cut them into thin strips. Scatter the mint strips over the brochettes and dust them with coarsely ground black pepper. Garnish with the remaining mint sprigs.

Serves 20 (2 brochettes per serving)

CTC	Total Carbs	Fiber	Total Fat	Sat Fat	Protein	Calories
4.30	4.61	.31	1.45	.01	1.63	36

roast beef "kisses" with chives

The rare roast beef that you find in most supermarket deli sections is generally very moist and is a great time-saver. Here it is used as a "wrapper" for cream cheese. Use any soft, flavored cream cheese you can find. I happen to like the vegetable or chive and onion varieties.

6   very thin slices rare roast beef (about 5 ounces)
¼   cup soft, flavored cream cheese
2   bunches fresh long chives

Cut each slice of roast beef in half lengthwise, then crosswise, to get 4 pieces. Place 1 teaspoon cream cheese in the center of each piece of roast beef. Fold the corners over each other to enclose the cheese. Turn each little packet over and use your hands to form each packet into a circular shape.

Cut 1 bunch of chives in half across the width and scatter them on a platter. Place the roast beef "kisses" on the bed of chives. Mince the remaining 1 bunch of chives as finely as possible and scatter them on top of the "kisses." Sprinkle each with a few grains of coarse salt and coarsely ground black pepper.

Serves 12 (2 "kisses" per serving)

nutritionist's note: Deli roast beef is a convenient carb-free food to keep in your fridge for noshing. A few slices will satisfy and contain only ½ gram of saturated fat and 35 calories per ounce.

CTC	Total Carbs	Fiber	Total Fat	Sat Fat	Protein	Calories
.68	.71	.03	2.65	1.77	2.76	39

little camembert popovers

These delectable, bite-size puffs act as warm pillows for chilled caviar. If you don't want to use salmon caviar, you can substitute sevruga, osetra, or beluga! Salmon caviar is the least expensive and the most colorful.

8	ounces Camembert cheese, chilled
3	extra-large eggs
¼	cup salmon caviar

Using a small, sharp knife, cut the rind from the cheese and discard the rind. Let the cheese sit at room temperature for 30 minutes.

Preheat the oven to 350°F.

In a food processor, place the eggs and process briefly. Cut the cheese into 1" pieces and add them to the processor. Process until very smooth and thick, about 1 minute.

Coat two 12-hole mini-muffin tins (about 1¼" in diameter) with cooking spray. Spoon 1 tablespoon of the cheese mixture into each cup. Bake for 10 to 11 minutes, until the popovers are slightly golden, puffed, and just firm to the touch. Remove the tins from the oven, let them sit for 1 minute, then remove the popovers by turning the muffin tins over. Top each warm or room-temperature popover with a dollop of caviar and serve.

Makes 24 (2 popovers per serving)

nutritionist's note: Caviar is a luxurious low-carb treat with only 1 gram of carbohydrates per ounce.

CTC	Total Carbs	Fiber	Total Fat	Sat Fat	Protein	Calories
.44	.44	0	5.64	2.76	5.68	74

crispy grape leaves with feta cheese

These attractive little packages pack a Mediterranean flavor wallop in just a few bites. Helen, my nutritionist, suggests several of these on a salad for a lovely low-carb lunch.

16	large grape leaves, packed in brine
8	ounces low-fat feta cheese
¼	cup extra-virgin olive oil

Separate the grape leaves and rinse them under cold water. Pat each one dry with paper towels. Cut each grape leaf in half from the tip down to the bottom through the stem. Remove the stems and any large veins.

Cut the cheese into rectangles, approximately 2" long by ¾" wide by ⅓" thick. Wrap each piece of cheese in a halved grape leaf, folding the sides in like an envelope and rolling up to cover the cheese completely.

In a large nonstick skillet over medium-high heat, heat the oil. Cook the wraps until the grape leaves become crispy and the cheese begins to melt, 1 to 2 minutes per side. Remove with a spatula to a serving platter and serve warm.

Serves 16 (2 pieces per serving)

CTC	Total Carbs	Fiber	Total Fat	Sat Fat	Protein	Calories
.70	1.14	.44	5.90	2.04	1.99	62

bombay shrimp

Serve these as hot and spicy as you'd like, tapas-style on little plates with small forks or toothpicks. Tandoori paste can be found in jars in some supermarkets, Indian markets, and specialty food stores.

36   medium shrimp in their shells (about 1 pound)
1   cup light coconut milk
4   teaspoons tandoori paste

Peel the shrimp. In a medium saucepan, place the shrimp shells and cold water to cover. Add 1 teaspoon salt and bring to a boil. Reduce the heat and simmer for 20 minutes. Strain the broth through a fine-mesh strainer and set aside.

In a small bowl, whisk together the coconut milk and tandoori paste until thoroughly blended. Pour into a nonstick skillet that is large enough to accommodate the shrimp in a single layer. Bring the mixture to a boil and add the shrimp. Cook, stirring often, until the shrimp turn opaque and just firm, 2 to 3 minutes. Remove the shrimp with a slotted spoon to a platter and cover with foil to keep warm.

Return the skillet to the heat and bring the sauce to a boil, adding a little shrimp broth to make it smooth. Boil until the sauce is very thick, 1 to 2 minutes. Add salt and pepper to taste, if needed, and pour over shrimp. Serve immediately.

Serves 6

nutritionist's note: Be certain to buy light coconut milk when cooking the low-carb and low-fat way. Almost none of the flavor is compromised.

CTC	Total Carbs	Fiber	Total Fat	Sat Fat	Protein	Calories
1.89	2.59	.70	3.23	2.18	8.89	74

chicken-pesto satays

Yum! These look great, and their heady fragrance of basil and garlic clearly announces their arrival. These can also be made with strips of pork, cut from a 5-ounce boneless pork chop. I've provided the nutritional data for both versions. You'll need 10 bamboo skewers to make these.

1	thick, skinless, boneless chicken breast (½ pound)
2	tablespoons prepared pesto
1	small clove garlic

Cut the chicken breast to get 10 long, thin strips that are about ⅛" thick and ½" wide. Thread each strip on a short bamboo skewer, weaving the skewer in and out of the chicken, like a ribbon. Try to cover as much of the skewer as possible so the skewers don't burn under the broiler.

In a small bowl, place the pesto. Squeeze the garlic through a garlic press and stir it into the pesto. Spread the pesto-garlic mixture on all sides of the chicken satays and sprinkle with salt and freshly ground black pepper. Cover and refrigerate for 3 to 4 hours to marinate.

When ready to serve, preheat the broiler.

Line up the satays on a rimmed metal baking sheet. Broil about 6" from the heat for 1 to 2 minutes. (Be careful not to overcook.) Serve immediately.

Serves 5 (2 skewers per serving)

chicken

CTC	Total Carbs	Fiber	Total Fat	Sat Fat	Protein	Calories
.33	.56	.23	1.65	.41	11.05	64

pork

CTC	Total Carbs	Fiber	Total Fat	Sat Fat	Protein	Calories
.33	.56	.23	2.69	.81	6.65	55

rosemary meatballs

It's amazing how moist low-fat turkey can taste, provided you don't overcook the meatballs. My husband loves these.

½   **pound lean ground turkey**
1   **small onion**
1   **small branch fresh rosemary**

In a medium bowl, place the turkey. Peel the onion and cut it in half. Grate the onion on the large holes of a box grater to get 2 tablespoons grated onion pulp and juice. Add the onion pulp and juice to the turkey.

Reserving some rosemary sprigs for garnish, remove the leaves from the rosemary and mince it as finely as possible to get 1 teaspoon. Add it to the turkey. Add a scant ½ teaspoon salt and ¼ teaspoon freshly ground black pepper to the turkey. Mix until all of the ingredients are incorporated. (You can continue at this point or cover the mixture and refrigerate it for up to 1 hour.)

Form the mixture into 16 meatballs. Heat a large nonstick skillet over high heat until hot. Add the meatballs and cook for 2 minutes. Reduce the heat to medium and roll the meatballs around the pan so they don't stick. Cook, turning the meatballs occasionally, until the meat is just firm, 3 to 4 minutes. (Do not overcook; you want them to remain moist.) Serve immediately, garnished with the reserved rosemary sprigs.

Serves 4 (4 meatballs per serving)

CTC	Total Carbs	Fiber	Total Fat	Sat Fat	Protein	Calories
.36	.47	.11	4.02	1.01	11.56	82

med-rim lamb patties

The easiest way to cook these is to form them into silver-dollar-size patties and sear them in a hot skillet. In the Middle Eastern style, however, you can pack the mixture onto bamboo skewers and broil them. Either way, they are delicious.

½ **pound lean ground lamb**
1 **small onion**
2 **teaspoons ground cumin**

In a small bowl, place the lamb. Peel the onion and cut it in half. Grate the onion on the large holes of a box grater to get 3 tablespoons grated onion pulp and juice. Add the onion and its juice to the lamb with the cumin, ½ teaspoon salt, and ¼ teaspoon freshly ground black pepper.

Using your hands, form the mixture into 12 meatballs, then press down on each ball to make a patty.

Heat a very large nonstick skillet over high heat until hot. Place the patties in the skillet and cook for 3 minutes. Turn them over and cook 2 minutes longer, or to the desired doneness. These can also be cooked under the broiler, until slightly charred. (Do not overcook. These are most flavorful and moist when they are slightly pink in the center.) Serve immediately.

Serves 6 (2 patties per serving)

nutritionist's note: Lamb is on the "occasional" list of diet programs that limit saturated fat. To guarantee that your ground lamb is lean, have your butcher grind it for you from the leanest cut available.

CTC	Total Carbs	Fiber	Total Fat	Sat Fat	Protein	Calories
.58	.74	.16	2.41	.82	8.07	59

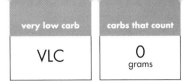

steak bits, buffalo-style

Buffalo-style refers to the famous chicken-wing dish from Buffalo, New York, where fried chicken wings are dipped into a mixture of Frank's Red Hot sauce and melted butter. If you substitute rare nuggets of steak, you will have an even better time. You can use top round (which is often used for London broil), sirloin steak, or a cut I love called chicken steaks. If you can't find Frank's Red Hot sauce or want even more heat, you can use Tabasco.

½   **pound top round steak, ½" thick**
2   **tablespoons butter**
2   **tablespoons Frank's Red Hot sauce**

Cut the steak into 20 cubes. In a very large skillet over high heat, briefly heat ½ tablespoon of the butter. Cook the meat in the butter until browned on the bottom, about 2 minutes. Turn it over and cook on the other side until browned, about 2 minutes longer. (Be sure to keep it rare.) Remove the steak from the heat and sprinkle it with salt.

Meanwhile, melt the remaining 1½ tablespoons butter and place it in a large bowl. Whisk in the hot sauce until incorporated.

With a slotted spoon, transfer the hot meat to the hot sauce–butter mixture. Toss quickly and, using a slotted spoon, transfer the meat to a plate. Serve with toothpicks with the remaining hot sauce–butter mixture in small bowls alongside for dipping.

Serves 4 (5 pieces per serving)

CTC	Total Carbs	Fiber	Total Fat	Sat Fat	Protein	Calories
.02	.06	.04	10.69	5.42	11.93	146

soups and starters

First courses was once a territory ruled by shrimp cocktails with high-sugar cocktail sauce and salads bathed in "carb-a-rator" dressings (sugar! fructose! corn syrup!), and hearty soups full of carbs (pasta! rice! corn starch! flour thickeners!). This chapter offers some of these old favorites in new, lovably low-carb guises. But in general, the soups and starters here embrace the trend toward food that is lighter, cleaner, more eclectic, more fun, and, of course, simple to prepare.

Adding a first course to any meal is a terrific way to get the family seated together for more than 10 minutes. You can hold a conversation about the food—or your day—instead of merely touching base. Or, if you're anything like me, you may opt to prepare two or three starters instead of a main course and call it dinner.

Three-ingredient soups are deliciously intriguing. Pay particularly close attention when purchasing their components: The freshness rule for all 1-2-3 recipes is especially important when it comes to soups. Anything less than fresh becomes glaringly apparent, so the best possible produce is essential—asparagus standing at stiff attention with tightly closed tips, unblemished peppers, ripe tomatoes, and herbs with their perfumes intact. My soups offer delightful textures as well as tastes, so you'll be using your blender or food processor fairly frequently and deploying some interesting techniques—like roasting vegetables for a thick tomato bisque or boiling zucchini as a base for a suave crab-flecked soup.

You may be surprised to find that soups using cream, half-and-half, and butter can be low carb, low cal *and* low in saturated fat. Small amounts of these choice fats have an exponential effect on richness and flavor. I've also learned that water, rather than stock, can help keep inherent flavors pristine.

Clear soups such as bouillons and consommés may be a bit old-fashioned, but I love to begin a meal with them as a kind of seduction. And while soup typically implies something warm and steamy, several of the recipes that follow are perfect for serving ice-cold on a sultry summer day.

Other starters in this chapter run the gamut from a generous Smoked Fish Plate with Lemon Cream Cheese (page 89) to tender Baby Spinach Salad with Crispy Bacon (page 101) to sizzling Lemon-Pepper Shrimp (page 100). In addition, many recipes from other sections in the book also make great first courses. From Party Food, try Bombay Shrimp (page 61), Steak Bits, Buffalo-Style (page 65), or Chicken-Pesto Satays (page 62). Other great options include halved portions of dishes from the Fish and Shellfish, Poultry, and Meat chapters—many of them with zero CTCs! From the Vegetables and Side Dishes chapter, who wouldn't love Poached Asparagus with Wasabi Butter (page 192) or Roasted Cauliflower with Cheddar Cheese (page 198) or Asiago-Roasted Fennel (page 202) as a prelude to a meal?

I encourage you to wander through and decide for yourself what a first course is!

chilled avocado soup

This surprising soup will have everyone guessing what's in it! Smooth, satiny, and very delicious, it is a chic way to begin a meal.

2   large ripe avocados
3   cups good-quality chicken broth
¼   cup dry sherry, preferably fino

Cut the avocados in half lengthwise, around the pits. Twist to split, then remove the pits and discard. Using a medium-size spoon, scoop out the flesh in large pieces, then cut into ½" pieces.

In a heavy medium saucepan, combine the broth and 2 cups water. Bring to a boil, then reduce the heat to a simmer. Add the avocado pieces and simmer for 2 minutes. Add 2 tablespoons of the sherry and cook 1 minute longer.

Remove the saucepan from the heat and let cool for several minutes. Transfer the contents of the saucepan to a blender. (You may need to do this in several batches.) Process until the soup is very smooth and creamy. Add salt and freshly ground white pepper to taste. Stir in the remaining 2 tablespoons sherry and chill until very cold before serving.

Serves 6

nutritionist's note: For years, avocado was seen as a high-fat demon, but it is angelic for a low-carb lifestyle: silky, filling, and high in heart-healthy monounsaturated fats.

CTC	Total Carbs	Fiber	Total Fat	Sat Fat	Protein	Calories
2.26	5.61	3.35	10.95	1.82	3.75	138

iced cucumber-yogurt soup

Kirby cucumbers, traditionally used to make pickles, are stubby and full of flavor. This soup is just as refreshing made with cilantro instead of mint.

1½   pounds kirby cucumbers
2   cups low-fat plain yogurt
1   bunch fresh spearmint or peppermint, finely chopped

Peel the cucumbers. Cut them in half lengthwise and use a small spoon to scoop out their seeds. Cut the cucumbers into ½" chunks.

Working in 2 batches if necessary, in a blender, combine the cucumbers, 1¾ cups of the yogurt, and 6 tablespoons of the chopped mint. Process until very, very smooth. Add kosher salt and freshly ground black pepper to taste. Cover and refrigerate for several hours—the colder the better. (The soup will thicken a bit.) Serve with a dollop of the remaining yogurt and garnish with chopped mint and coarsely ground black pepper.

Serves 4

nutritionist's note: Buy extra kirby cucumbers to keep on hand for a crunchy, low-carb snack. One cup of peeled, sliced cucumbers has only 2 grams CTC.

CTC	Total Carbs	Fiber	Total Fat	Sat Fat	Protein	Calories
10.99	12.48	1.49	2.10	1.22	7.21	94

roasted yellow pepper-tomato bisque

Slowly roasting the vegetables and then pureeing them provides one set of taste experiences, while the chopped raw vegetables added later provide contrast. It is delicious served cold, gazpacho-style, or hot.

6	large ripe tomatoes (about 2 pounds)
3	large yellow bell peppers (about 1½ pounds)
2	tablespoons + 2 teaspoons basil-flavored oil

Preheat the oven to 300°F.

Remove the cores from 5 of the tomatoes. Cut them in half through the stem ends and place them in a large bowl. Cut 2 of the peppers in half lengthwise. Remove the stems, any thick interior ribs, and seeds and discard. Place the peppers in the bowl with the tomatoes. Pour 1 tablespoon of the oil over the vegetables. Sprinkle with 1½ teaspoons salt and coarsely ground black pepper. Toss to coat thoroughly.

Place the tomatoes and peppers, cut sides down, on a rimmed baking sheet. Roast for 1 hour. Turn the vegetables over and roast for another hour. Turn them over again and roast for an additional 30 minutes. (The total roasting time is 2½ hours.)

Transfer the vegetables to a food processor. Add 1½ cups boiling water to the baking sheet. Using a spatula, scrape up all the browned bits and accumulated juices. Add the liquid and browned bits to the food processor. Process until very smooth. Transfer the soup to a large bowl. Whisk in 1 tablespoon of the oil and salt and freshly ground black pepper to taste. Refrigerate the soup for several hours until very cold. Add more water if it seems too thick and adjust the seasonings as needed.

Cut the remaining tomato in half horizontally. Squeeze out the seeds and discard them. Cut the remaining tomato flesh into tiny cubes. Remove the stems, any thick interior ribs, and seeds from the remaining pepper and finely dice it. Scatter the diced vegetables over each serving of soup and drizzle with the remaining 2 teaspoons oil.

Serves 4

nutritionist's note: This recipe's added health bonus is that the carb-free basil oil helps your body to absorb the beta-carotene in the peppers. The soup is also high in desirable fiber.

CTC	Total Carbs	Fiber	Total Fat	Sat Fat	Protein	Calories
15.56	21.46	5.90	10.07	1.37	3.44	173

ginger and chicken consommé

There is a Chinese proverb that says, "He who cooks simplest cooks best." This soup is a fine example. A homeopathic doctor might prescribe this highly restorative soup for whatever ails you, including a minor case of the blues.

6   cups low-sodium chicken broth, organic if possible
5   scallions
1   4" piece fresh ginger

In a heavy medium saucepan, place the broth. Bring just to a boil, then reduce the heat to medium.

Coarsely chop 4 of the scallions, including half of the dark green parts. Reserve about 3" of the remaining dark green part for later and discard the rest. Add the chopped scallions to the broth. Cook until the broth is reduced to about 4 cups, 20 to 25 minutes. Strain the soup through a fine-mesh sieve into a clean saucepan.

Peel the ginger and grate it on the large holes of a box grater. Place the grated ginger in a paper towel and squeeze the juice into a small bowl. Discard the grated ginger. Very thinly slice the remaining scallion and reserved 3" of the dark green parts on the bias and add it to the soup along with the ginger juice. Cook for 2 minutes, then add salt and freshly ground black pepper to taste, if needed. Serve immediately.

Serves 4

CTC	Total Carbs	Fiber	Total Fat	Sat Fat	Protein	Calories
3.41	4.51	1.10	2.14	.59	8.04	71

madeira-beef bouillon

Back in the old days, clear soups made with port, Madeira, or sherry invariably were found on menus of fancy restaurants. They signaled sophistication and lightness and were an elegant way to begin a meal. I've added a layer of flavor with a bit of prosciutto. If you're serving this as an inter-mezzo between courses, you might want to eliminate the prosciutto and instead slip a very thin slice of lemon into each soup bowl or elegant cup.

6   cups good-quality, low-sodium beef broth
1   slice (2 ounces) prosciutto, about ⅛" thick
½   cup Madeira

In a medium saucepan, combine the broth and 1 teaspoon black peppercorns. Bring to a boil, then reduce the heat and cook until the broth is reduced to about 4 cups, about 20 minutes.

Meanwhile, cut the prosciutto into very thin strips and set it aside at room temperature.

Add the Madeira to the soup and bring it to a boil. Reduce the heat and simmer for 2 minutes. Add a pinch of salt; the prosciutto will add additional salty flavor. Ladle immediately, leaving the peppercorns behind, into shallow soup bowls and evenly distribute the prosciutto. Serve immediately.

Serves 4

CTC	Total Carbs	Fiber	Total Fat	Sat Fat	Protein	Calories
2.00	2.00	0	3.00	1.25	7.00	90

miso soup with chorizo

In just 5 minutes, you can serve this mysterious soup to your guests. They will have no idea what they're eating but will lap up every drop. White miso, which you can find in the refrigerated section of Asian markets and health food stores, is the secret ingredient, adding a winey background flavor. Smoked chorizo is available in most supermarkets these days.

6   baby bok choy (about 6 ounces)
3   tablespoons white miso
3   ounces smoked Spanish chorizo sausage

Cut the bok choy lengthwise into thin strips and set it aside.

In a medium saucepan, combine 4 cups cold water and the miso. Whisking constantly, cook the mixture over medium heat until very hot, making sure it doesn't boil. Lower the heat and simmer for 2 minutes, add the bok choy, and cook until it is just tender, taking care not to overcook, about 2 minutes longer. Add a pinch of salt and freshly ground black pepper to taste.

Slice the chorizo into paper-thin slices on the bias. Add the chorizo to the soup and cook for 1 minute more. Ladle the soup into bowls and serve immediately.

Serves 4

nutritionist's note: Rapidly boiling miso can deplete its nutritional value, so heat it only until it is hot, or just below the boiling point.

CTC	Total Carbs	Fiber	Total Fat	Sat Fat	Protein	Calories
3.91	4.61	.70	8.98	3.17	7.25	126

garlic soup with chicken and cilantro

You can adjust the intensity of the garlic at the end by pressing more garlic through a press. Be sure to use an entire bunch of cilantro because its perfume will balance the garlic's. Note that this recipe requires advance preparation to allow the broth to cool.

5	pounds chicken wings
1	large bulb garlic
1	large bunch fresh cilantro

Cut the chicken wings in half, through the large joint, and place in a 6-quart pot along with 10 cups cold water. Cut the bulb of garlic in half crosswise and add it to the pot. Chop off the cilantro stems and add the stems to the pot. Reserve the cilantro leaves. Add 1 tablespoon salt and 1 teaspoon black peppercorns. Bring to a rapid boil, then reduce the heat to maintain a simmer and skim the foam from the surface. Cover and simmer for 2 hours.

Strain the soup through a fine-mesh sieve into a clean pot. Press down on the solids to extract all of the juices. (You will have about 10 cups broth.) Reserve the cooked chicken wings. Let the broth and chicken cool, then refrigerate until cold.

Skim off all of the fat from the cold broth. Heat just until boiling, lower the heat to medium, and cook, uncovered, until the liquid is reduced to 8 cups, about 30 minutes. (For a stronger garlic taste, add an additional clove of garlic, pushed through a press, during the final cooking.) Add salt to taste.

Meanwhile, pick the chicken meat from the wings and discard the bones and skin. Place the meat in a sieve and dip it into the hot broth to warm. Place about ¼ cup warmed chicken in the center of each of 8 shallow soup bowls. Tear the reserved cilantro leaves and divide among the soup bowls to taste. Pour 1 cup hot broth into each bowl and serve.

Serves 8

nutritionist's note: It has been well documented in scientific literature that garlic has beneficial properties that help maintain a healthy heart by lowering blood pressure and cholesterol.

CTC	Total Carbs	Fiber	Total Fat	Sat Fat	Protein	Calories
1.55	1.61	.06	2.46	.68	19.36	113

jade zucchini soup with crab

Serve this hot or cold. The soup's stunning jade color comes from pureed green zucchini skins. It is practically fat-free, yet it tastes remarkably rich. The better the crab, the better the soup, so avoid watery frozen crabmeat and spring for fresh lump crab bought at a good fish market.

1½   **pounds zucchini**
1   **bunch fresh dill**
½   **pound jumbo lump crabmeat**

Trim the ends of the zucchini and cut it into ½" pieces. Transfer the zucchini to a medium-large saucepan with a cover. Finely chop the dill to yield ¼ cup, reserving some dill sprigs for garnish. Add the dill to the saucepan with the zucchini.

Pick over the crab, making sure to remove any pieces of shell or cartilage. Place half the crab and any accumulated juices from the crab in the saucepan. Cover with 1½ cups water and add 1 teaspoon salt. Bring the liquid to a boil. Reduce the heat to a simmer, cover the pot, and cook until the zucchini is very soft, about 20 minutes. Remove from the heat and let cool for 5 minutes. Transfer the contents of the saucepan to a blender and process until very smooth. (This will take several minutes, and the soup will thicken to a foamy texture.) Add salt and freshly ground black pepper to taste. Transfer the soup back to the saucepan. Heat gently until hot, then ladle the soup into warm bowls and top with small mounds of the remaining crab. Garnish with sprigs of the remaining dill.

Serves 4

CTC	Total Carbs	Fiber	Total Fat	Sat Fat	Protein	Calories
2.95	5.01	2.06	.86	.18	12.23	73

broccoli soup with basil butter

You want to use really fresh basil here, and lots of it, because this aromatic herb flavors the broth, then perfumes the compound butter that floats on top. Because it's pureed, the soup appears rich and filling despite its low carb and calorie counts. For a really great presentation, use a small, sharp knife to cut off the tiny buds on top of the broccoli and scatter them on the soup before serving.

1	large bunch broccoli (about 1½ pounds)
1	large bunch fresh basil
4	tablespoons (½ stick) unsalted butter

Using a vegetable peeler, peel the broccoli stalks, removing the tough exterior. Cut off and discard the woody bottoms. Cut the broccoli stalks and florets into ½" pieces and transfer them to a medium pot.

Remove and reserve the smallest leaves of basil for garnish. Add ½ cup tightly packed basil leaves to the broccoli. Cover with 5 cups cold water and ½ teaspoon salt. Bring to a boil. Reduce the heat to medium, cover the pot, and cook until the broccoli is tender, about 20 minutes.

Meanwhile, place the butter and ¼ cup packed basil leaves in a food processor. Add a large pinch of salt and process until just combined. Scoop the butter onto a piece of waxed paper and roll to form a log about ½" in diameter. Refrigerate until firm.

When the broccoli is tender, transfer it to a blender using a slotted spoon. Add 2 cups of the cooking water, reserving the rest. Process until very smooth, about 2 minutes, adding 2 tablespoons basil butter in small bits as you process. (You may need to do this in several batches.) When the mixture is very smooth, return it to the pot. Add salt and freshly ground black pepper to taste. If it seems too thick, mix in some of the reserved cooking water.

Heat the mixture gently. Ladle the hot soup into soup cups or bowls. Place a thin slice of basil butter on top and garnish with the reserved small basil leaves. Serve immediately.

Serves 6

nutritionist's note: This recipe is a good example of using butter in a responsible way, keeping saturated fat within guidelines and keeping calories extremely low, while maintaining a high flavor profile.

CTC	Total Carbs	Fiber	Total Fat	Sat Fat	Protein	Calories
2.56	6.06	3.50	8.09	4.84	3.52	100

sweet garlic-fennel soup

When low-carbotarians who also are vegetarians come to dinner, I usually prepare this soup. It reminds me of luxurious oyster bisque and is every bit as special. In fact, the velvety richness and moderate calorie count may amaze you. And don't worry, the copious amounts of garlic merely thicken and sweeten the soup to perfection.

24   large cloves garlic
2   cups half-and-half
2   large fennel bulbs (about 1 pound each)

Cut the garlic cloves in half lengthwise and peel them. Remove and discard any woody ends and green shoots. Transfer the garlic to a 4-quart pot with a cover. Add the half-and-half, 4 cups water, and 1 tablespoon salt. Bring to a rapid boil. Reduce the heat to low, cover the pot, and simmer until the garlic is very soft, about 30 minutes.

Trim the wispy fronds from the fennel, finely chop them, and set aside. Cut away and discard all but 1" of the fennel stalks. Cut the fennel bulbs into ½" pieces, removing any brown spots. Wash in a colander under cold water and pat dry with paper towels.

Add the fennel to the pot. Add 2 tablespoons of the chopped fennel fronds to the pot with some ground white pepper. Bring to a boil, then reduce the heat to a simmer. Cover and simmer until the fennel is very soft, about 30 minutes.

In several batches, transfer the soup to a blender and process until very, very smooth. Return the soup to the pot and add salt and white pepper to taste. Heat gently and ladle into soup bowls. Garnish with the rest of the reserved chopped fennel fronds and serve immediately.

Serves 8

nutritionist's note: Soups like this traditionally call for heavy cream, but half-and-half allows an ultracreamy soup to fit into our specs for low saturated fat.

CTC	Total Carbs	Fiber	Total Fat	Sat Fat	Protein	Calories
11.74	15.55	3.81	7.24	4.33	4.10	135

creamy carrot-ginger soup

Sometimes carrots can be a good thing, even for carb counters. You'll be amazed how easy it is to extract the fresh ginger juice needed in this recipe and how perfectly its flavor melds with carrots. Heavy cream makes this soup taste luxurious.

1½   **pounds carrots**
1   **5" piece fresh ginger**
4½   **tablespoons heavy cream**

Trim the carrots, peel them using a vegetable peeler, and cut them into 1" pieces. Transfer the carrots to a medium-size pot and add 4 cups water and 1½ teaspoons salt. Bring to a boil, then reduce the heat and cook, uncovered, until the carrots are very soft, about 35 minutes.

Meanwhile, peel the ginger and grate it on the large holes of a box grater. Wrap the ginger in a paper towel and squeeze hard to extract juice. (You will have about 1 tablespoon juice.) Discard the grated ginger.

Transfer the carrots to a food processor and puree until very smooth, slowly adding all the cooking water as you process. Add the ginger juice and heavy cream and process to incorporate.

Return the soup to the pot and add salt and freshly ground black pepper to taste. Heat through and serve.

Serves 4

nutritionist's note: Carrots, formerly forbidden on low-carb plans, became acceptable in limited amounts when it was realized that their glycemic load was less taxing than originally thought. Eating carrots in moderation adds beneficial nutrients to one's overall diet.

CTC	Total Carbs	Fiber	Total Fat	Sat Fat	Protein	Calories
12.68	17.79	5.11	6.57	3.94	2.11	132

fresh asparagus soup

Asparagus and truffle oil—what could be more sophisticated? Their bouquets complement each other in fascinating ways. White truffle oil may be expensive, but a little bit goes an extraordinarily long way. You can buy it in small bottles in many supermarkets and most specialty food stores. Make this soup at the first whiff of spring.

2¼ **pounds medium asparagus**
3 **tablespoons unsalted butter**
2 **teaspoons white truffle oil**

Trim the woody ends from the bottoms of the asparagus stalks and discard them. Remove the tip plus 1" of the stalk from 8 asparagus spears. Transfer the 8 asparagus tips to a medium skillet (large enough for the spears to fit without crowding) with just enough water to cover. Bring to a boil, and cook for 2 minutes. Drain and set aside.

Using a vegetable peeler, peel the remaining asparagus spears plus the 8 bottoms, using a light touch. Cut the asparagus into 1" pieces. Place them in a large saucepan with a cover and add 1½ cups water, all but 1 teaspoon of the butter, and a large pinch of salt. Bring to a boil, then reduce the heat to medium. Cover the pan and cook until the tip of a small, sharp knife glides through the asparagus, about 8 minutes. (They should be yielding, but not too soft.)

Remove the saucepan from the heat and let it cool for 5 minutes. Transfer the asparagus and cooking liquid to a blender. Start the blender on low speed and gradually increase to high, pureeing until the soup is very, very smooth, 5 to 7 minutes. Transfer the mixture to a clean saucepan and add the truffle oil. Gently heat and add salt and freshly ground black pepper to taste.

In a small nonstick skillet over high heat, place the remaining 1 teaspoon butter and cook the reserved asparagus tips until hot and lightly browned, about 2 minutes. Ladle the hot soup into bowls, garnish with the asparagus tips, and serve.

Serves 4

CTC	Total Carbs	Fiber	Total Fat	Sat Fat	Protein	Calories
6.23	11.59	5.36	11.40	5.65	5.91	155

cream of cauliflower

Scallions are important here for reasons of both gastronomy and science. In addition to imparting their subtle flavor to the cauliflower, the pureed scallions add a lovely smoothness, and the dark greens make a welcome garnish. If served cold, this soup tastes like vichyssoise without carb-laden potatoes.

1   large or 2 small heads cauliflower (about 2½ pounds)
2   bunches scallions
1   cup light cream

Trim the base of the cauliflower, removing the stems and any dark spots. Break the cauliflower into small florets. Transfer the florets to a medium saucepan. Add 5 cups water and ½ teaspoon salt. (The water will not cover the cauliflower.) Trim the scallions and cut the white and light green parts into ¼" pieces, reserving the dark green parts. Add the chopped scallions to the pot with the cauliflower.

Bring the mixture to a boil, then reduce the heat to a simmer. Cover the pot and cook until the cauliflower is very soft, about 25 minutes. In batches if necessary, transfer the soup to a food processor and process until ultra-smooth, gradually adding the cream. Transfer the soup to a clean saucepan.

Reheat the soup, add salt and freshly ground black pepper to taste, and add a little water to thin, if necessary. Ladle into warm soup bowls. Slice the reserved dark green scallion parts into very thin slices on the bias or coarsely chop and sprinkle them liberally on the soup. Serve immediately.

Serves 6

nutritionist's note: The cruciferous cauliflower is a low-carb chameleon. By using it instead of potatoes, you save 20 CTC and still enjoy the ultracreamy texture.

CTC	Total Carbs	Fiber	Total Fat	Sat Fat	Protein	Calories
7.36	12.12	4.76	8.11	4.87	4.75	128

butternut bisque with crispy bacon

You'll want to make this vibrant soup during autumn and winter when butternut squash is in season. Roasting squash before simmering it into a soup intensifies the flavors and colors. Buy good-quality, nitrite-free bacon because it is an integral component of the soup's hearty appeal. It flavors the broth and adds crunch at the end.

1   large butternut squash (about 2 pounds)
1   pound medium leeks
8   slices nitrite-free bacon

Preheat the oven to 400°F.

Cut the squash in half across its width. Cut these pieces in half lengthwise. Place the squash, cut sides down, on a rimmed baking sheet and pour ½ cup water over the squash. Roast for 50 minutes, moving the pieces around with a spatula after 30 minutes so they don't stick. Remove the squash from the oven and set aside.

Cut the leeks into ½" pieces, using the white and light green parts and only 1" of the dark green parts. Wash the leeks well under running water in a colander, making sure to remove all the dirt. Pat very dry with paper towels. Set aside.

Cut 6 slices of the bacon into ½" pieces and add to a 4-quart pot. Cook over high heat, stirring constantly to release some of the fat, for 1 minute. Add the chopped leeks to the pot with the bacon, reduce the heat to medium, and cook, stirring often, until the leeks are well softened and beginning to color, about 10 minutes.

Scoop out the flesh from the squash shells and add it to the pot with the leeks. Add 3 cups water and ½ teaspoon salt to the pot and bring to a boil. Reduce the heat to a simmer, cover the pot, and cook for 20 minutes. In two batches, transfer the soup to a blender. Process until very smooth and velvety. Add salt and freshly ground black pepper to taste. Return the soup to the pot and reheat gently before serving. Add some water if it seems too thick.

Meanwhile, in a small skillet over medium heat, cook the 2 remaining slices of bacon until crisp. Drain and discard the fat. Pat the bacon dry with paper towels, coarsely crumble it, scatter it on the soup, and serve.

Serves 6

CTC	Total Carbs	Fiber	Total Fat	Sat Fat	Protein	Calories
18	20.88	2.88	8.29	2.71	7.16	177

cold oysters with hot sausages

This is a classic pairing of cold and hot, salty and spicy tastes. Chipolata, sometimes called little fingers, are highly spiced pork sausages, about 2 to 3 inches long. You may substitute small breakfast links or even Vienna sausages, or you could make my Homemade Turkey Sausage (page 38) and roll them into little "fingers." You can find chipolata in some butcher shops and specialty food stores.

20   large oysters, freshly shucked, on the half shell

12   small chipolata sausages or 8 breakfast links

1   lemon, cut into wedges

On each of 4 large plates, place a bed of coarse salt. Place 5 oysters on each plate.

In a skillet over medium-high heat, cook the sausages until browned and piping hot, about 3 minutes. Blot the sausages with a paper towel to remove excess fat and serve them immediately alongside the oysters with thin wedges of lemon.

Serves 4

CTC	Total Carbs	Fiber	Total Fat	Sat Fat	Protein	Calories
3.74	3.74	0	11.77	4.05	10.21	165

cherrystone clams
with white balsamic mignonette

Mignonette sauce is a French invention, but I've substituted more mellow white balsamic vinegar for a softer balance of sweetness and acidity. You can grind your own black peppercorns very coarsely or buy cracked black or mignonette peppercorns in a jar.

32   cherrystone clams
½   cup white balsamic vinegar
4   shallots

Open the clams, keeping them on the half shell. (You can have your fishmonger do this for you, if desired.) Cover the clams and refrigerate them until ready to use.

In a small bowl, stir together the vinegar and 2 tablespoons cold water. Peel the shallots and very finely mince them to get 2 heaping tablespoons. Add the shallots to the vinegar with 1 tablespoon very coarsely ground black pepper and a pinch of salt and stir to combine. (If the mignonette sauce tastes too sharp, you can add a little more cold water.)

For each serving, place 8 clams on a bed of crushed ice or on a bed of coarse salt. Serve with small bowls of the mignonette sauce for dipping.

Serves 4

CTC	Total Carbs	Fiber	Total Fat	Sat Fat	Protein	Calories
8.66	8.66	0	1.14	.11	15.07	113

chilled shrimp cocktail
with low-carb cocktail sauce

The secret to making really great-tasting shrimp is to cook them and cool them in water that's as salty as the sea. Most cocktail sauces are carb-laden, but this version is clean and spicy and has far fewer carbs.

30   large shrimp in their shells (about 1 1/2 pounds)

1 2/3   cups V8 juice

1/3   cup prepared white horseradish

Bring a large pot of water to a rapid boil. Add lots of salt. Add the shrimp, reduce the heat to medium, and cook until the shrimp are just firm, 3 to 4 minutes. (Do not overcook.) Immediately transfer the shrimp into a bowl of ice-cold, heavily salted water to cool. Peel the shrimp, leaving the tails intact. Wrap the shrimp well and refrigerate them until ready to serve.

In a small, nonreactive saucepan, bring the V8 juice to a boil. Reduce the heat to medium and cook, stirring occasionally, until it is reduced to 1 cup, 10 to 15 minutes. Let cool. Stir in the horseradish and chill until cold.

Serve 5 shrimp per person on a bed of ice with small bowls of the cocktail sauce for dipping.

Serves 6

CTC	Total Carbs	Fiber	Total Fat	Sat Fat	Protein	Calories
6.02	6.30	.28	4.37	.32	22.90	129

boiled lobster with wasabi mayonnaise

Half of a chilled lobster is a sublime way to begin a low-carb meal. The wasabi mayo is addictive and also great with crab claws, cold shrimp, or chilled mussels. You'll find wasabi powder in specialty food stores and in the Asian section of most supermarkets.

2   lobsters (1½ pounds each)
2½ tablespoons wasabi powder
⅔   cup light mayonnaise

In a very large pot with a cover, combine 10 quarts water and enough salt to make the water taste salty. (The pot should be filled three-quarters of the way to the top.) Cover the pot and bring the water to a rapid boil.

Add the lobsters, one at a time. Bring the water back to a rapid boil. After the water returns to a boil, reduce the heat to medium and cover the pot. Cook for 15 to 18 minutes. Remove the lobsters from the pot with tongs and transfer them to a colander. Set them under cold running water until they cool. Refrigerate the lobsters until they are very cold.

Meanwhile, in a small bowl, combine the wasabi powder and 2 tablespoons cold water and stir to make a paste. Stir in the mayonnaise and mix until the ingredients are thoroughly blended. Add a pinch of salt and stir. Cover the mixture and refrigerate it until cold.

When ready to serve, split the lobsters in half lengthwise through the heads, cutting down in one swift movement through the tails. Crack the claws across the width of the claw with a swift hit with the back of a large, heavy knife. Serve half a lobster on each serving plate with a small bowl of wasabi mayonnaise for dipping.

Serves 4

nutritionist's note: Using light mayonnaise instead of regular mayonnaise keeps the CTC controlled and cuts the saturated fat in half.

CTC	Total Carbs	Fiber	Total Fat	Sat Fat	Protein	Calories
4.28	4.65	.37	14.69	2.93	26.77	266

avocado and crab "martini"

Here is comfort food redefined: jumbo lump crab and avocado presented in a chilled martini glass. Ripe avocado and fresh lime juice are whirled into a rich, velvety sauce that blankets the crab. Buy the best crabmeat you can find and make your fishmonger swear to its freshness. Alongside a small salad, this is substantial enough for lunch.

14 ounces fresh jumbo lump crabmeat
2 small ripe avocados
3 limes

Chill 4 large martini or wine glasses in the freezer.

Pick through the crabmeat to remove and discard any shells or cartilage. Set the crabmeat aside.

Cut the avocados in half lengthwise around the pits. Twist to separate the sides and remove the pits. Using a small, sharp knife, remove the skin of 2 halves. Cut the flesh into small pieces, between ¼" and ½", and transfer to a small bowl. Cut 1 lime in half and squeeze some lime juice over the chopped avocado to prevent discoloration. Add salt and freshly ground black pepper and gently toss.

Scoop out the avocado flesh from the remaining 2 halves. Add it to a food processor along with 2 tablespoons fresh lime juice (squeezed from 1 lime), ⅓ cup cold water, and salt and freshly ground black pepper to taste. Process until very smooth and thick.

To serve, fill the chilled glasses with some of the lime-marinated chopped avocado. Top with the crab-meat and spoon the avocado sauce over the crabmeat. Garnish with slices or wedges of the remaining lime. Dust with coarsely cracked black pepper and serve.

Serves 4

CTC	Total Carbs	Fiber	Total Fat	Sat Fat	Protein	Calories
3.73	8.06	4.33	16.06	2.46	19.38	244

peppered tuna "tataki"

This Japanese-inspired dish has become popular in restaurants, so why not try making it at home? Buy a piece of top-quality tuna that is log-shaped, similar to a filet mignon, or a thick tuna steak that weighs 1 pound. It's cooked briefly, just to sear the tuna on all sides, and the center stays sushi-style "raw." Be sure to use roasted peanut oil for an extra layer of flavor. It is available in many supermarkets, Asian markets, and specialty food stores.

2	tablespoons roasted peanut oil
1	pound best-quality fresh tuna, in 1 piece
¼	cup balsamic vinegar

Brush 1 tablespoon of the peanut oil all over the tuna. Finely crush 3 tablespoons black peppercorns and press them all over the surface of the tuna. Sprinkle the tuna lightly with salt.

Set a large nonstick skillet over high heat until it's very hot. Quickly sear the tuna on all sides so that only the outer area of the fish gets cooked, about 20 seconds per side. (The inside will be almost raw.) Transfer the tuna to a cutting board to cool.

Meanwhile, in a small nonstick skillet, bring the vinegar to a boil. Boil for 1 to 2 minutes, until reduced to 2 tablespoons. Remove from the heat and let cool for 5 minutes. Mix the reduced vinegar with the remaining 1 tablespoon roasted peanut oil and a pinch of salt.

With a very sharp knife, cut the tuna into paper-thin slices and arrange them on 4 large plates. Drizzle each plate with some of the vinegar-oil mixture.

Serves 4

nutritionist's note: Roasted peanut oil is a great choice for this recipe because it can withstand the high heat required for searing the tuna, it is carb free (many people mistakenly assume peanut oil has carbs), and it is a good source of heart-healthy monounsaturated fat

CTC	Total Carbs	Fiber	Total Fat	Sat Fat	Protein	Calories
2.00	2.00	0	12.31	2.57	26.46	233

smoked fish plate with lemon cream cheese

This is one of the simplest and perhaps most satisfying ways to begin a meal for company. Trading up a bit to purchase the best quality smoked salmon, sturgeon, or sable makes all the difference in the success of this dish. You can also serve store-bought gravlax, which can be found in most gourmet food stores.

12   ounces smoked fish (salmon, sturgeon, or sable), thinly sliced
6   tablespoons whipped cream cheese
2   lemons

On each of 4 large plates, lay out the fish slices in slightly overlapping fashion.

In a medium bowl, place the cream cheese. Grate the zest of 1 lemon and add half of the zest to the cream cheese. Halve the lemon and add 1 teaspoon lemon juice to the cream cheese. Using a fork, beat it together until creamy.

Serve the fish with a dollop of lemon cream cheese in the center. Scatter the remaining lemon zest over the cheese. Serve with thin wedges of the remaining lemon.

Serves 4

CTC	Total Carbs	Fiber	Total Fat	Sat Fat	Protein	Calories
.19	.35	.16	12.00	5.75	19.53	181

prosciutto e melone

Done in the true Italian style, gossamer slices of slightly salty prosciutto form a coverlet for slightly sweet slices of cantaloupe. Shards of Parmesan cheese—try to buy real Parmigiano-Reggiano—add a nutty contrast. Pass the pepper mill at the table. Instead of prosciutto, you may substitute speck, which is smoked prosciutto and is available at Italian specialty food stores and some supermarkets.

½   ripe cantaloupe
½   pound imported prosciutto, very thinly sliced
2   ounces Parmesan cheese, in one piece

Using a small, sharp knife, remove the rind from the cantaloupe. Cut the cantaloupe into very thin slices and arrange it in the centers of 4 large plates in slightly overlapping patterns. Add a grinding of black pepper. Drape the prosciutto over the melon to cover it completely.

Using a small, sharp knife or cheese slicer, cut paper-thin shards of cheese, scatter it over the prosciutto, and serve.

Serves 4

nutritionist's note: Prosciutto is a great example of a food that provides high-impact flavor, yet it is carb free and has only 1 gram of saturated fat per ounce.

CTC	Total Carbs	Fiber	Total Fat	Sat Fat	Protein	Calories
5.75	6.30	.55	10.45	4.75	22.50	209

carpaccio of beef with mustard mayonnaise

This low-carb, raw beef dish is a carnivore's dream that's readily found in restaurants but hardly ever at home. It's actually easy to make. Buy the meat the same day you're going to serve it. Have your butcher slice the raw meat paper-thin, or you can freeze the meat slightly and, using a sharp, thin-bladed knife, slice it yourself. If you don't like the idea of raw meat, you can sear the beef lightly in a skillet and quickly chill it, making certain it is still very rare in the center. You can use cooked roast beef from the supermarket, but only if it is very rare.

6	tablespoons light mayonnaise
3	tablespoons Dijon mustard
1	pound top round of beef or boneless beef tenderloin, sliced paper-thin

In a small bowl, whisk together the mayonnaise and mustard, adding a pinch of salt, if necessary.

When ready to serve, arrange the beef slices in an overlapping fashion on 6 large, chilled plates. For a decorative touch, put the mustard-mayonnaise in a small squeeze bottle and squeeze it in a decorative pattern over the beef. Or dip a fork in the mustard-mayonnaise and carefully drip the sauce in lines across the beef. Season with coarse sea salt and coarsely ground black pepper and serve.

Serves 6

CTC	Total Carbs	Fiber	Total Fat	Sat Fat	Protein	Calories
1.67	1.81	.14	8.52	2.04	17.71	159

roast turkey tonnato

Traditionally a veal dish made during the summer in Italy, tonnato refers to a refreshing sauce with tuna brightened with lemon. To save the bother of roasting veal, I've used turkey breast instead, which is readily available in most any market. Just make sure you're getting freshly roasted turkey breast, not the packaged stuff that's pumped full of water and chemicals. This is also a lovely main course for a light lunch. It's delicious with the Beefsteak Tomato and Sweet Onion Salad (page 94).

1   can (6 ounces) light tuna packed in olive oil
2   lemons
1   pound roast turkey breast, sliced ⅛" thick

In a blender, place the tuna with its oil. Grate the zest of both lemons so that you have 2 teaspoons zest. Squeeze the lemons to get ¼ cup juice. Add 1 teaspoon of the grated zest to the blender with the lemon juice. Puree until very, very smooth, adding a little cold water, if necessary. Add salt and freshly ground black pepper to taste and blend. Cover and refrigerate until cold.

When ready to serve, arrange the turkey slices on 4 large plates. Drizzle the tonnato dressing over the turkey. Scatter the remaining lemon zest on top and pass the pepper mill at the table.

Serves 4

CTC	Total Carbs	Fiber	Total Fat	Sat Fat	Protein	Calories
3.12	3.29	.17	15.39	2.50	30.54	271

chilled asparagus with creamy sesame dressing

This yummy Middle Eastern–inspired dressing with its bracing background of lemon juice and zest has great affinity for chilled asparagus. You'll find jars of tahini—ground sesame seeds—in specialty food shops, health food stores, or the ethnic food aisle at most supermarkets. Add some fresh garlic to lemony tahini, and you've got a perfect 1-2-3 sauce for grilled chicken or fish.

1½   pounds medium asparagus
2   lemons
½   cup tahini

Cut 1" from the bottom of the asparagus stalks and discard. Peel the lower half of the stalks with a vegetable peeler. Bring a large pot of salted water to a boil. Add the asparagus and cook over medium-high heat until they are bright green and tender, about 5 minutes. (Be careful not to over-cook.) Drain the asparagus immediately and plunge it into a bowl of ice water to prevent further cooking. Remove the asparagus from the water and pat it dry with paper towels. Wrap the asparagus in plastic and refrigerate until ready to serve.

Grate the zest of the lemons and set aside. Cut both lemons in half and squeeze to get 6 tablespoons juice.

Stir the tahini in the jar, making sure to incorporate any oil that may have risen to the top. Place ½ cup tahini in a food processor. Begin to process, adding the lemon juice and 5 to 6 tablespoons water until you have a smooth, thick puree. Add salt and freshly ground black pepper to taste. Stir in the lemon zest. Cover and refrigerate until cold.

When ready to serve, divide the cold asparagus among 6 chilled plates. Spoon the tahini sauce over the midsections of the asparagus. Pass the pepper mill at the table.

Serves 6

CTC	Total Carbs	Fiber	Total Fat	Sat Fat	Protein	Calories
7.10	11.32	4.22	9.80	1.39	5.82	141

beefsteak tomato and sweet onion salad

Instead of the sweet sticky dressing usually associated with this steakhouse salad, I use my very best (and most expensive) extra-virgin olive oil. You may substitute another oil if you please, such as basil-, lemon-, garlic-, or citrus-flavored oil.

2   medium sweet onions, such as Vidalia
4   ripe medium beefsteak tomatoes (about 2 pounds)
¼   cup extra-virgin olive oil

Peel the onions and slice them ⅛" thick. Remove the cores from the tomatoes and slice them ¼" thick. Transfer several slices of the tomato (about ½ tomato) to a blender and process with a pinch of salt until smooth.

On 4 large, chilled plates, alternate sliced tomatoes and onions, arranged in a circle or in a straight line. Drizzle with the oil and the tomato puree. Sprinkle with coarse salt and very coarsely ground black pepper and serve.

Serves 4

nutritionist's note: Barry Kimmel, MD, a prominent urologist, tells his low-carbing male patients to include lots of tomatoes in their diets to maintain prostate health. "When men cut carbs," Dr. Kimmel says, "they tend to cut down on healthy fruits and vegetables."

CTC	Total Carbs	Fiber	Total Fat	Sat Fat	Protein	Calories
11.79	15.27	3.48	14.34	1.94	2.56	188

mesclun with lemon-raspberry vinaigrette

Because it is so light, this salad of fancy greens makes the perfect starter for a substantial meal or it can be a simple lunch when paired with one of my low-carb soups. Thankfully mixed mesclun greens are available in most supermarkets. Using a good-quality raspberry vinegar from France is your best bet because cheap versions are often sweetened.

5   ounces mesclun greens
3   tablespoons raspberry wine vinegar
⅓   cup lemon-flavored olive oil

Chill the greens until ready to use.

In a small bowl, place the vinegar and, using a small wire whisk, slowly whisk in the oil until well blended. Add salt and freshly ground black pepper to taste.

In a large serving bowl, place the chilled mesclun greens. Add the dressing and quickly toss, coating the leaves thoroughly. Add a bit of salt and pepper to taste, if necessary. Serve immediately.

Serves 4

CTC	Total Carbs	Fiber	Total Fat	Sat Fat	Protein	Calories
1.22	1.57	.35	18.08	2.44	.46	168

bibb lettuce and roasted pepper salad with creamy feta dressing

Here's a salad that's so robust I often serve it alongside a grilled steak and eliminate the veggies entirely! If you appreciate bitterness, substitute well-washed chicory leaves for the Bibb lettuce.

4   large bell peppers, 2 red and 2 yellow
5   ounces feta cheese
2   medium-large heads Bibb lettuce

Preheat the broiler.

Put the peppers on a rimmed baking sheet and broil them for several minutes on each side, about 6" from the heat, until the skins are very black and blistered. Immediately transfer the peppers to a paper bag, close tightly, and let them sit to steam for 10 minutes. You can also put them in a bowl and cover it with a tightly fitting lid.

Remove the peppers and carefully peel or scrape away all of the charred skin. Place the peppers on a platter. Cut the peppers in half and remove the cores and seeds, carefully collecting any juices that accumulate. Let the peppers cool, then cut into ⅓"-wide strips.

Into a food processor, crumble the cheese. Process until very smooth and thick, gradually adding up to ½ cup cold water. Add freshly ground black pepper and blend.

Break the lettuce into large pieces and place a mound on each of 4 large plates. Top with roasted pepper strips and all of the accumulated juices. Drizzle with the feta dressing. Add a grinding of coarsely ground black pepper and serve.

Serves 4

CTC	Total Carbs	Fiber	Total Fat	Sat Fat	Protein	Calories
9.65	13.64	3.99	8.01	5.36	7.41	147

seared salmon on lemony cucumbers

In this pretty dish, salmon is cooked from the bottom up so that the fish gets progressively rarer toward the top. There's an interesting contrast of textures and temperatures between the chilled, crunchy cucumbers and the warm, yielding fish. Hothouse cucumbers are the more expensive, seedless variety, sold in most better supermarkets.

1   pound hothouse cucumbers
2½   tablespoons lemon-flavored olive oil
4   salmon fillets (4 ounces each), without skin

Peel the cucumbers. Slice the cucumbers into paper-thin rounds and toss them in a colander with 2 teaspoons coarse salt. Weight down the cucumbers with a bowl and place the colander in a larger bowl or in the sink to catch the liquid. Let sit for 1 hour, then wash off the salt under cold running water. Press the cucumbers between your hands to extract as much liquid as possible. Toss the cucumbers with 1 tablespoon of the oil and season with freshly ground black pepper. Chill until ready to serve.

In a nonstick skillet over medium-high heat, add ½ tablespoon of the oil. Heat until just hot and add the salmon. Cook for 3 minutes. (The bottom of the salmon will get crisp and the top quarter will still be uncooked.) Cover the skillet and cook until the top just beings to turn opaque, about 2 minutes longer. (Do not overcook.) Uncover, remove from the heat, and sprinkle the salmon with salt. Let the salmon cool to room temperature, if desired.

When ready to serve, mound the cucumbers in the center of 4 medium-large plates. Top each mound with a piece of warm or room-temperature salmon. Drizzle with the remaining 1 tablespoon oil and serve.

Serves 4

CTC	Total Carbs	Fiber	Total Fat	Sat Fat	Protein	Calories
1.53	2.13	.60	15.76	2.29	22.98	246

chardonnay mussels

This dish employs an interesting technique that allows the mussels to open in a hot, dry pan in the oven, which imparts a subtle flavor. I use Chardonnay for its full-bodied, slightly oaky finish, but Japanese sake or a "grassy" Sauvignon Blanc would also be good choices.

2	pounds medium-large mussels
1	large bunch fresh cilantro
¾	cup oaky chardonnay, from California or Australia

Preheat the oven to 500°F.

Place a large cast-iron skillet in the oven until it is very hot, about 15 minutes.

Scrub the mussels, removing the beards, if any. When the skillet is hot, remove it from the oven using an oven mitt or pot holder because the handle will be dangerously hot. Carefully add the mussels to the skillet and return it to the oven. Roast for 6 to 8 minutes, until the mussels have opened.

Meanwhile, coarsely chop the cilantro to get 1 cup.

Again using an oven mitt or pot holder, remove the skillet from the oven and place it on the stove top over high heat. Pour the wine over the mussels and add ¾ cup of the chopped cilantro. Cook until some of the alcohol evaporates, about 2 minutes. Divide the mussels equally among 4 large flat soup bowls. Top with the remaining chopped cilantro.

Serves 4

CTC	Total Carbs	Fiber	Total Fat	Sat Fat	Protein	Calories
4.47	4.96	.49	2.34	.44	12.29	121

mussels à la marinara

Briny juices from steamed mussels coalesce with the flavors of fennel and tomato in this dish. The flavors will remind you of a beach vacation. Fennel has two roles: It becomes the chunky textural component of the dish, and its fronds are a graceful garnish.

2	pounds medium-size mussels
1	cup good-quality marinara sauce
1	medium fennel bulb, with lots of feathery fronds

Scrub the mussels, removing the beards, if any.

In a medium pot with a cover, combine the marinara sauce with 1¾ cups water. Remove the stalks with fronds from the fennel bulb. Finely chop the fennel fronds and set them aside. Discard the stalks or save them for another use.

Cut the fennel bulb in half lengthwise and then crosswise into paper-thin slices. Add the fennel to the pot with a large pinch of salt and ½ teaspoon cracked black pepper or more to taste. Bring to a rapid boil, then reduce the heat to medium and cook until the fennel is just tender, about 8 minutes.

Add the mussels to the pot and quickly cover. Increase the heat to high and cook until the mussels open, about 6 minutes. Shake the pot back and forth to evenly distribute the mussels. Discard any mussels that haven't opened, then, using a slotted spoon, transfer the opened mussels to 4 large bowls or flat soup plates. Raise the heat to high and cook the sauce for 1 minute to thicken a bit. Immediately spoon the sauce over the mussels. Scatter the chopped fennel fronds on top and serve immediately.

Serves 4

nutritionist's note: Carbohydrate levels vary significantly among different brands of marinara sauce, so be sure to read the nutrition labels carefully and buy one without added sugar or corn sweeteners and under 5 grams of carbohydrates per ½ cup.

CTC	Total Carbs	Fiber	Total Fat	Sat Fat	Protein	Calories
10.17	12.93	2.76	3.62	.61	13.39	138

lemon-pepper shrimp

Once upon a time, I poured this dish over pasta, but that was before the low-carb revolution, when I discovered it was good enough to eat on its own. The lemons soften during cooking and are meant to be eaten along with the shrimp. This recipe calls for thin-skinned lemons; choose lemons that give slightly when squeezed.

20   jumbo shrimp in their shells (about 1¼ pounds)
2   thin-skinned lemons
3½   tablespoons extra-virgin olive oil

Peel and devein the shrimp and pat them dry with paper towels. Thinly slice the lemons and remove any seeds.

In a very large nonstick skillet, heat the oil over high heat until it is hot. Add the shrimp and lemon slices and cook, stirring constantly, for 2 minutes. Add 2 teaspoons coarsely cracked black peppercorns. Continue to cook, stirring over high heat, until the shrimp has turned opaque, about 2 minutes longer. (Be careful not to overcook the shrimp.) Add salt to taste.

Immediately transfer the shrimp, lemons, and pan juices to 4 plates. Serve immediately.

Serves 4

CTC	Total Carbs	Fiber	Total Fat	Sat Fat	Protein	Calories
4.54	7.08	2.54	14.41	2.07	29.42	265

baby spinach salad with crispy bacon

This sumptuous, but simply made, salad is also delicious with arugula. It is best to prepare this salad right before you are going to serve, otherwise the leaves will wilt.

6   ounces fresh baby spinach
8   slices nitrite-free bacon
3   tablespoons white balsamic vinegar

Place the spinach in a bowl.

Cut the bacon into ½"-wide pieces. In a large nonstick skillet over medium-high heat, cook the bacon until it gets crispy, but not too crisp, and all of the fat is rendered. When the bacon is cooked, quickly remove it with a slotted spoon and let it drain on paper towels, reserving the fat in the skillet.

Add the vinegar and a large pinch of salt to the bacon fat in the skillet and cook over medium heat, stirring constantly, for 1 minute. Remove the skillet from the heat and let cool for 1 minute. Pour enough dressing over the spinach to coat, but not saturate, the leaves and toss. Add freshly ground black pepper and salt, if needed.

Quickly divide the mixture among 4 large plates and top with the cooked bacon. Serve immediately.

Serves 4

CTC	Total Carbs	Fiber	Total Fat	Sat Fat	Protein	Calories
1.84	2.99	1.15	12.15	4.02	9.22	157

meat

Unlimited portions of char-grilled sirloin, 2"-thick pork chops, ½-pound burgers blanketed with cheese, and all the bacon you want—these are the images that hooked many Americans on the idea of low-carb diets. The idea, however tenuous and controversial, that we could eat these things with wild abandon seemed to satisfy our most primal urges and started a revolution that celery never could.

After the revolution comes the revelation: No one should indulge in unlimited quantities of meat. The calories really add up, and, more importantly, so does the saturated fat, which has been shown to clog arteries, raise cholesterol, and even lead to heart disease.

The point of *Low Carb 1-2-3* is to eat not dogmatically, but well. That means eating sensibly, eating simply, and eating lots of different things. Dietary goals that are based on unrealistic portions are doomed to failure—few people will ever be satisfied by a puny 3-ounce portion of meat. *Low Carb 1-2-3* portions are more realistic and more generous, yet they still fit into one of our low-carb categories, and they never contain more than 6 grams of saturated fat per serving.

And look at what you have to choose from to keep your low-carb meals interesting: Braised Hoisin Pork with Scallions (page 109), Pesto-Crusted Rack of Lamb (page 113), Sun-Dried Tomato Meat Loaf (page 117), *Tournedos au Poivre* with Balsamic Syrup (page 121), and Broiled Veal Steak with Fresh Thyme Mustard (page 129). This is certainly not your father's meat and potatoes!

Some of the recipes can be prepared a day in advance; in the case of slow-braised meats, an extra day in the fridge can improve flavors. Other meats require only a quick flash-cooking in a hot pan.

Either way, the essence of foolproof meat cookery is to apply the proper technique to the right cut of meat and then serve it at the proper degree of doneness. Fundamentally, you cook meat either quickly at high temperature or at a leisurely pace at low temperature.

High-heat cookery—grilling a pork chop or searing a steak—creates Americans' favored charred and caramelized exterior, leaving a slightly chewy interior. These methods are great for backyard barbecuing or for getting dinner on the table quickly. Be sure to season steaks and chops well—with salt and pepper—before *and* after cooking for optimal flavor.

And then there's slow cooking, in which you envelop your meat with moist heat that transforms less expensive hunks of pork, lamb, or veal into spoon-tender braises and stews that are bathed in lip-smacking natural juices.

My objective is to achieve depth of flavor. Recent studies show that boosting flavors actually reduces hunger. You don't need to eat *a lot* to feel satisfied, just *well*.

parmesan-crusted pork tenderloins

This is an unusual combination of flavors, but they really work together. The cheese forms a handsome crust around the pork, helping to seal in the juices. If you're bashful about cumin, feel free to use ground sage instead.

2	pork tenderloins (14 ounces each)
¾	cup freshly grated Parmesan cheese, about 3 ounces
2	tablespoons ground cumin

Preheat the oven to 375°F.

Pat the pork dry with paper towels and lightly season it with salt.

In a small bowl, mix together the cheese, cumin, and freshly ground black pepper to taste. Press the mixture all over the pork, coating it as thoroughly as possible.

Place the pork on a rimmed baking sheet or in a shallow roasting pan. Bake for 12 minutes. Turn the pork over and bake for 10 minutes longer. (The pork should be slightly pink in the center.) Remove the pork from the oven, transfer it to a cutting board, and let it rest for several minutes before serving. Cut the pork into ½"-thick slices and serve immediately.

Serves 4

CTC	Total Carbs	Fiber	Total Fat	Sat Fat	Protein	Calories
0	1.20	1.20	13.75	6.04	50.70	339

sausage-and-fruit-stuffed pork

This is a great holiday dish without any fuss. It will look as spectacular as anything you'll see on the cover of a food magazine. Here a little dried fruit goes a long way in satisfying sweet cravings and provides a great contrast to the slightly salty sausage.

8   ounces turkey sausage
2   ounces dried mixed fruit
2½ pounds boneless center-cut pork loin

Preheat the oven to 375°F.

Spray a shallow roasting pan or rimmed baking sheet with cooking spray.

Remove the sausage from the casings and crumble it into a bowl. Cut the fruit into ¼" dice, add it to the sausage, and mix together.

Make a slit down the middle of the entire length of the pork, making sure to leave the bottom half uncut. Season the resulting channel with salt and freshly ground black pepper. Fill the pork with the sausage mixture, packing it in tightly. Using kitchen string, tightly tie the pork at ½" intervals, then wrap the string once around the length of the pork.

Season the pork with salt and black pepper and place the pork, cut side down, on the prepared roasting pan or baking sheet. Roast for about 25 minutes, then turn the pork over. Roast for 30 minutes longer, or until the temperature on an instant-read thermometer reaches 150°F. Transfer the pork to a cutting board.

Add ½ cup boiling water to the pan juices and scrape up any browned bits. Strain the liquid through a sieve into a saucepan. Add salt to taste and cook over high heat for a few minutes to thicken. Carve the pork into thick slices and serve with the pan juices.

Serves 6

nutritionist's note: The rule for eating dried fruit on most low-carb plans is to limit consumption or eat only occasionally. In this recipe, you get only ⅓ ounce per serving, which is limited indeed.

CTC	Total Carbs	Fiber	Total Fat	Sat Fat	Protein	Calories
6.82	8.82	2.00	18.95	5.37	41.52	364

brined pork loin with dry sherry

Immersing pork in a bath of salt water before roasting keeps it juicy without adding perceptible saltiness. Roasted peanut oil and dry sherry add a fragrant air of sophistication.

2   pounds boneless pork loin, tied with kitchen string at ½" intervals
2   tablespoons roasted peanut oil
¾   cup dry sherry

In a large bowl, combine 8 cups water and ¼ cup kosher salt and stir to dissolve. Add the pork. Add more water if necessary to cover the pork. Cover and refrigerate for 4 to 6 hours. Remove the pork from the brine and pat dry with paper towels.

Preheat the oven to 400°F.

In a large baking dish with a cover, heat 1½ tablespoons of the oil over medium-high heat. Add the pork and quickly brown on all sides. Place the browned pork on a rimmed baking sheet. Roast the pork for 30 minutes, or until the temperature on an instant-read thermometer reaches 150°F. Transfer the pork to a cutting board and let it rest while you prepare the sauce.

In a small saucepan, combine the sherry and ¼ cup water and bring to a boil. Add the sherry mixture to the baking sheet and scrape up any browned bits. Strain the juices through a fine-mesh sieve back into the saucepan. Add the remaining ½ tablespoon oil and bring to a boil. Cook over high heat until the liquid is reduced by half. Add 1 teaspoon coarsely ground black pepper and salt to taste. Cut the pork into ⅓" slices and serve hot with the sauce.

Serves 6

CTC	Total Carbs	Fiber	Total Fat	Sat Fat	Protein	Calories
1.75	1.75	0	15.52	4.96	28.76	291

garlic-miso pork chops

I've become addicted to using white miso, also known as shiro miso, to deeply flavor all kinds of protein. It makes a great marinade for pork chops, imparting an indefinable taste and very moist texture. For the brave of palate, you can finely chop an extra clove of garlic and sprinkle it on the chops before serving. You can find shiro miso in Asian food markets, health food stores, and many supermarkets.

¼ cup white miso
3 medium cloves garlic
4 center-cut thick pork chops (8 ounces each)

Up to 1 day before you plan to serve, in a small bowl, mix together the miso and 1 tablespoon water. Press the garlic through a garlic press, add it to the miso, and mix well. Thickly spread the miso mixture on all sides of the pork. Put the pork in a shallow baking dish large enough to hold the pork in 1 layer and cover with foil. Marinate, refrigerated, for 8 to 12 hours, turning several times.

When you're ready to cook the pork, preheat the broiler.

Remove the pork from the baking dish and evenly respread the miso marinade over the chops. Place the pork on a rimmed baking sheet. Lightly dust the pork with freshly ground black pepper. Place the pork under the broiler, 4" to 5" from the heat, and broil for 5 minutes. Turn the pork over and broil 5 minutes longer. Remove the pork from the oven and serve immediately.

Serves 4

CTC	Total Carbs	Fiber	Total Fat	Sat Fat	Protein	Calories
4.11	5.16	1.05	17.17	6.05	33.63	309

braised hoisin pork with scallions

Lip-smacking and luscious, this dish is deeply flavored and only vaguely Asian. Hoisin sauce, a sort of Chinese-spiced ketchup but more complex, is one of my requisite pantry staples.

2	bunches scallions (about 4 ounces)
1	boneless pork shoulder (5 pounds)
6	tablespoons hoisin sauce

Preheat the oven to 300°F.

Trim the roots from the scallions. Cut on the bias into 1" lengths, using the white and green parts.

Leave a little fat on the pork, trimming away all the rest. If the pork has not already been tied when you bought it, roll the pork tightly and, using kitchen string, tie in 2" intervals. Heat a very large baking dish with a cover over high heat until very hot. Add the pork, fatty side down, and brown for a few minutes. Then turn the pork and brown it on all sides for a total of 10 minutes of cooking time. Remove from the heat. While the pork is still in the pan, spread the hoisin sauce over the pork. Scatter the scallions over the pork and add 1 teaspoon black peppercorns. Cover the pot and bake for 3½ hours, or until the pork is very tender.

Transfer the pork and scallions to a cutting board. Using a large spoon, remove as much fat as possible from the pan juices and place the baking dish on top of the stove. Cook the liquid over high heat until very reduced and syrupy, adding salt and freshly ground black pepper to taste.

Lightly sprinkle the pork with salt and cut it into thick slices. Scatter with the scallions, pour the hot sauce over top, and serve.

Serves 6 (about 7 ounces per person)

nutritionist's note: A little hoisin sauce can fit into your low-carb life. Hoisin provides about 6 CTC per serving and lots of satisfying flavor.

CTC	Total Carbs	Fiber	Total Fat	Sat Fat	Protein	Calories
7.56	8.50	.94	16.46	5.57	39.3	349

st. patrick's day pork and cabbage

This authentic recipe, known as "Irish bacon," is traditional St. Patrick's Day fare in Ireland—never corned beef. Brined pork simmered with lots of garlic and cabbage produces amazingly succulent meat. This is a substantial, Sunday kind of supper. Serve it with very spicy mustard.

1   pork shoulder or Boston butt (7 pounds), with bone
3–4 very large bulbs garlic (about 6 ounces)
1   large head green cabbage (about 2 pounds)

One day before you plan to serve, trim the pork of almost all its fat. Place the pork in a very large pot. Dissolve 3 cups kosher salt in 1 gallon water and pour over the pork to cover, adding more water if needed. Cover the pot and refrigerate for 24 hours.

Bring the pork and brine to a boil. Boil 10 minutes and then drain the pork thoroughly. Add enough fresh water to the pot to cover the pork and bring to a rapid boil.

Cut the garlic bulbs in half through their equators and add the garlic to the pot with ½ tablespoon black peppercorns. Cover the pot and cook over medium-low heat for 3 hours, about 25 minutes per pound, or until the pork is very tender. Remove the pork from the pot and place it in a large shallow baking dish. Cover to keep warm.

Cut the cabbage into 6 wedges and add them to the pot. Bring the water to a boil and cook until the cabbage is soft, about 20 minutes. Remove the cabbage and garlic with a slotted spoon and place on a large platter. (Note that most of the garlic will have dissolved into the broth.) Lightly sprinkle the cabbage with salt. Cut the pork into thick pieces and place alongside the cabbage. Ladle hot broth over the pork and serve.

Serves 8 (approximately 7 ounces per serving)

CTC	Total Carbs	Fiber	Total Fat	Sat Fat	Protein	Calories
10.14	13.19	3.05	14.58	4.96	41.78	354

pork shoulder with garlic-thyme crust

People who only prepare pork chops or loins miss out on the homespun fun of the shoulder. This cut is juicier, more flavorful, and less formal. In this recipe, I gradually raise the oven temperature to guarantee a crunchy, crackling crust.

1   pork shoulder (5 pounds)
2   large bunches fresh thyme
12 large cloves garlic

Preheat the oven to 350°F.

Trim most of the fat from the pork shoulder. Chop the fat into very small pieces to make ⅓ cup. Remove enough leaves from the thyme to get ⅓ packed cup. Set aside any remaining thyme branches.

Press 4 cloves of the garlic through a garlic press and rub the garlic all over the pork shoulder. Mince the remaining 8 cloves garlic. Chop the garlic with the thyme leaves, pork fat, and 1 teaspoon coarse salt to make a paste. Make ¼"-wide, 1"-deep holes all over the pork and fill them with the garlic-thyme mixture. Also insert the mixture around the bone. (The idea is to infuse the flesh with as much flavor as possible.)

Put the remaining thyme branches in the bottom of a roasting pan or large shallow baking dish. Place the pork on top of the branches. Roast for 45 minutes, then increase the oven temperature to 400°F and roast for 25 minutes longer. Increase the heat again to 450°F and roast for an additional 25 minutes, or until the temperature on an instant-read thermometer reaches 145°F. Transfer the pork to a cutting board, let rest for 10 minutes before carving, carve as desired, and serve.

Serves 6 (approximately 7 ounces per serving)

CTC	Total Carbs	Fiber	Total Fat	Sat Fat	Protein	Calories
3.15	3.65	.50	14.25	4.92	39.51	310

baby lamb chops with english mint sauce

Once upon a time, when lamb was gamier tasting, the Brits served it with a savory mint sauce, while Americans served it with emerald green mint jelly. My version has a touch of sweetness from sea-soned rice vinegar and speckles of fresh mint. It is more in tune with today's lamb, which is milder. Seasoned rice vinegar is rice vinegar with salt and sugar added. It is still within our low-carb guide-lines. It is available in supermarkets and Asian food stores.

¾	cup seasoned rice vinegar, chilled
1	bunch fresh mint
12	rib lamb chops

In a small bowl, place the vinegar. Finely chop enough mint to get ¼ cup and combine the mint with the vinegar. Reserve the remaining mint to use as a garnish. Add a pinch of salt and freshly ground black pepper to the vinegar and stir to mix. Set aside the vinegar mixture in the refrigerator.

Preheat the broiler.

Season the lamb with salt and pepper. Place the lamb on a broiler pan. Broil the lamb for 4 minutes on each side, or until it reaches the desired doneness.

Sprinkle the lamb again with salt and serve immediately, garnished with the reserved sprigs of fresh mint and served with the chilled mint sauce.

Serves 4 (3 chops per serving)

nutritionist's note: It is possible to use seasoned rice vinegar, which has some added sweetener, if it is in moderation.

CTC	Total Carbs	Fiber	Total Fat	Sat Fat	Protein	Calories
12.03	12.06	.03	15.71	5.62	34.00	333

pesto-crusted rack of lamb

I've snuck a single slice of whole wheat bread into this recipe to hold the pesto sauce atop the lamb, but fear not, we're still in the low-carb zone. This makes for a very elegant and extremely easy candle-light dinner for two.

1   slice whole wheat bread
1   8-rib rack of lamb, trimmed, flap removed, and bones exposed
⅓   cup good-quality prepared pesto

Preheat the oven to 375°F.

To make bread crumbs, lightly toast the bread, let it cool, tear it into pieces, and process it to crumbs in a food processor. Put the crumbs in a metal baking dish and bake for 10 minutes, shaking once, to dry them out.

Season the lamb with salt and freshly ground black pepper. Spread the pesto over the surface of the lamb. Thoroughly coat the pesto-rubbed lamb with the bread crumbs, lightly packing them down with your hands. Cover the exposed bones with foil and place the lamb, bread crumb side up, on a baking sheet.

Roast the lamb for 15 minutes, remove the foil, and bake for 20 minutes longer. Remove the lamb from the oven, let it rest for 5 minutes, and dust it lightly with salt. Slice the lamb into thick double chops or single chops and serve immediately.

Serves 2

nutritionist's note: When choosing prepared pesto, buy the brand that has the lowest fat content. Also check your nutrition labels when buying whole wheat bread. Make sure it does not contain added sugar, honey, or corn syrup.

CTC	Total Carbs	Fiber	Total Fat	Sat Fat	Protein	Calories
6.29	8.81	2.52	15	4.82	39.38	336

slow-braised lamb in merlot

This recipe thumbs its nose at today's school of high-speed cooking. Cooking the lamb for 5 hours results in meltingly tender meat, and copious amounts of garlic cloves give up their sting in favor of heady perfume. You make this all in one pot, and all the recipe asks for is time.

1	boned leg of lamb (4 pounds)
1	bottle Merlot or other sturdy dry red wine
40	large cloves garlic

Up to 1 day before you plan to serve, with a very sharp knife, cut away and discard most of the lamb's fat. Tightly roll the lamb and, using kitchen string, tie it at 1″ intervals. Select a heavy casserole with a cover large enough to hold the lamb. Put the lamb in the casserole and pour in all but ½ cup of the wine. Lightly crush all but 1 clove of the garlic and remove the skins. Place the garlic in the casserole. Cover and refrigerate for 8 hours.

Preheat the oven to 300°F.

Remove the casserole from the refrigerator and add 1 teaspoon whole black peppercorns. Set the casserole on the stove top and bring to a boil, uncovered, skimming off some of the foam that rises to the surface. Cover the casserole and put it in the oven. Cook for 1 hour. Turn the lamb over and cook for 3½ hours longer, or until spoon-tender, turning once or twice again during cooking

Remove the lamb from the casserole. With a large spoon, remove as much fat as possible from the pan juices. Add the remaining ½ cup wine and 1 clove garlic, pushed through a garlic press. Over high heat, boil the pan juices until reduced by half. Add a generous amount of salt and freshly ground black pepper. Remove from the heat. Slice the lamb and add it to the pot. Let the lamb absorb the juices. Warm gently, if necessary, before serving.

Serves 6 (approximately 6 ounces of lamb plus sauce per serving)

CTC	Total Carbs	Fiber	Total Fat	Sat Fat	Protein	Calories
8.31	8.73	.42	11.86	4.52	41.73	397

spiced lamb with ginger and cilantro

Geographically speaking, this dish could come from Southeast Asia or from the Middle East. But in truth it tastes only like itself, because the cooking process melds these 3 distinct ingredients into a new flavor dimension.

2   large bunches fresh cilantro
1   6" piece fresh ginger (about 5 ounces)
1   leg of lamb (4½ pounds), butt half, bone in

Up to 1 day before you plan to serve, remove the leaves from 1 bunch of the cilantro and put them in a food processor.

Using a small, sharp knife, peel the ginger. Cut the ginger into large chunks and add to the food processor with the cilantro. Add 1 teaspoon coarse salt and ½ teaspoon cracked black pepper. Process until a coarse paste forms. (Do not overprocess because you don't want the result to be watery.)

Rub the ginger-cilantro mixture over the lamb. Tightly pack some on top of the lamb to form a thick layer. Place the lamb in a large plastic bag and secure it tightly. Refrigerate for 8 hours.

Remove the lamb from the refrigerator and let it sit at room temperature for 30 minutes before cooking. Meanwhile, preheat the oven to 375°F.

Using a sharp knife, lightly score the top of the lamb with lines 1" apart. Place the lamb in a heavy, shallow roasting pan and roast for about 18 minutes per pound, or until the temperature on an instant-read thermometer reaches 145°F for medium-rare. You may need to drain the fat halfway through cooking. Transfer the lamb to a cutting board, let it rest for 5 minutes, and carve it as desired.

Serve immediately, garnished with fresh cilantro sprigs from the remaining 1 bunch cilantro.

Serves 6 (approximately 6 ounces per serving)

CTC	Total Carbs	Fiber	Total Fat	Sat Fat	Protein	Calories
2.62	3.11	.49	14.72	5.73	40.26	318

smokey joe burgers

If you haven't been inclined to hunt down a source for smoked paprika, this recipe will be your motivation. It will also become your family's favorite burger. A little grated onion adds untold amounts of moisture and flavor. These can be pan-seared, broiled, or cooked on the grill. Smoked paprika, from Spain, can be found in specialty food stores and many supermarkets.

2   pounds ground sirloin
1   medium onion
2   teaspoons smoked paprika

About 3 hours before you plan to serve, place the sirloin in a large bowl. Halve the onion through the equator. Grate the onion halves on the large holes of a box grater to yield 2½ tablespoons onion pulp. Add the onion pulp to the sirloin. Add the smoked paprika and 1 teaspoon salt to the bowl. Using your hands, mix the ingredients to incorporate thoroughly. (Do not overwork the mixture.)

Shape the meat into 6 large, thick patties. Individually wrap each burger in foil. Refrigerate for 3 hours, but no longer, to let the flavors mingle.

Preheat the broiler.

Put the burgers on a rimmed baking sheet and broil, about 6" from the heat, for 3 to 4 minutes on each side until they reach the desired doneness. (Do not overcook.) Serve immediately.

Serves 6

CTC	Total Carbs	Fiber	Total Fat	Sat Fat	Protein	Calories
1.49	1.97	.48	10.86	4.03	31.76	240

sun-dried tomato meat loaf

Meat loaf recipes are often haphazard accumulations of way too many ingredients, but this version rolls things back to the fundamental few. Ice cubes—my mother's secret—keep the meat moist and juicy. You can also shape the meat into burgers and sear them in a skillet.

1   cup sun-dried tomatoes in olive oil
1   medium-large onion
1½   pounds ground sirloin

Preheat the oven to 350°F.

Drain the oil from the sun-dried tomatoes into a large nonstick skillet. Finely dice the tomatoes and set them aside.

Finely dice the onion to get 1 packed cup. Set the skillet over medium heat and add the diced onion. Cook slowly, stirring occasionally, until the onion is soft and golden, about 10 minutes.

In a large bowl, combine the sirloin, diced tomatoes, cooked onion with all the pan juices, 1 teaspoon salt, and freshly ground black pepper.

In a bowl, combine ¼ cup cold water and 3 slightly crushed ice cubes and add to the sirloin. Mix thoroughly. Shape into an 8″ × 4½″ loaf and place on a rimmed baking sheet or in a shallow roasting pan. Bake for 35 to 40 minutes. Remove the sirloin from the oven and let rest 5 minutes before serving.

Serves 4

CTC	Total Carbs	Fiber	Total Fat	Sat Fat	Protein	Calories
7.56	9.87	2.31	16.17	5.12	37.15	335

arthur schwartz's stracetti

Arthur Schwartz, author of Naples at Table, *is one of the world's foremost experts on Italian cuisine. He also knows how to make simple things taste divine. This is his 3-ingredient adaptation of a beloved Italian beef dish known as stracetti, which means "rags." Serve this atop a mound of bitter greens, as he does, or just with a fork and knife, as I do.*

¼   cup rosemary-flavored olive oil
3   large cloves garlic, lightly smashed
1   pound filet mignon, sliced ¼" thick

In a large skillet, combine the oil and garlic. Place over low heat and cook slowly to let the oil infuse with the garlic, about 2 minutes. (The garlic should get soft, but not colored.) Press the garlic into the oil with the back of a wooden spoon to release its flavor. (This can be done hours ahead.) Before cooking the meat, remove the garlic and discard.

Pound the filet into very thin rounds. Have the butcher do this for you or use a flat meat pounder, not a tenderizer, to do it yourself. Lightly season the filet with salt and freshly ground black pepper.

Place the skillet with the seasoned oil over high heat. When the oil is hot but not smoking, gradually add the slices of filet to the pan, and cook for about 15 seconds per side. As the meat is done, arrange it in overlapping slices on a warm platter. When all the meat has been cooked, pour the oil and pan juices over the meat. Sprinkle with coarse salt and coarsely ground black pepper and serve immediately.

Serves 4

CTC	Total Carbs	Fiber	Total Fat	Sat Fat	Protein	Calories
.93	.99	.06	23.55	5.90	23.75	316

double-garlic skirt steak

Skirt steak, although a bit chewy, is perhaps the most flavorful cut of beef and stands up to the bold amount of garlic—used roasted and raw—in this recipe. For those new to salsa verde, it is a green sauce made from tomatillos instead of tomatoes and can be found in jars in the Mexican food sections of better supermarkets.

2	very large bulbs + 4 large cloves garlic
2	skirt steaks (12 ounces each)
2	cups prepared medium-hot salsa verde

Up to 1 day before you plan to serve, preheat the oven to 400°F.

Loosely wrap 2 bulbs of the garlic in aluminum foil. Place them in a small baking dish and roast for 1 hour. Remove from the oven and let cool.

In a large bowl, combine the steak and 1½ cups of the salsa verde. Cut the roasted garlic bulbs in half crosswise and squeeze out the soft garlic pulp. Add the garlic to the bowl. Slice the raw garlic cloves lengthwise into paper-thin slices. Add to the bowl and mix the ingredients thoroughly. Cover and refrigerate a minimum of 6 hours, or overnight.

Remove the steaks from the marinade and cut each steak into 2 portions. Discard the leftover marinade.

Heat 1 very large or 2 smaller nonstick skillets over high heat. Place the steaks in the hot pans and cook to the desired doneness, 3 to 5 minutes on each side. (You want the steak blackened and caramelized on the outside and rare inside.) Sprinkle with coarse salt and freshly ground black pepper. Cut on the bias into ¼" slices and serve with the remaining ½ cup salsa verde.

Serves 4

nutritionist's note: Salsa verde is an excellent source of vitamin C. The discarded marinade is subtracted from the total amount of salsa to calculate how much is consumed in the recipe.

CTC	Total Carbs	Fiber	Total Fat	Sat Fat	Protein	Calories
9.16	10.36	1.20	13.61	5.84	35.09	319

pot roast with smothered red onions

Sometimes doing nothing is sufficient. In this recipe, there's no browning or sautéeing. You just put the ingredients into a pot and let them, quite literally, stew in their own juices. And like many "potted" dishes, it tastes even better the next day.

2   pounds red onions
1   rump or chuck roast (3 pounds)
1   cup dry vermouth

Preheat the oven to 275°F.

Cut the onions in half through the stem ends. Place the cut sides down on a cutting board and thinly slice the onions across the width. Put the onions in a large ovenproof pot with a cover. (An enameled cast-iron Le Crueset pot is very good for this.)

Season the roast with salt and freshly ground black pepper and place it on the onions in the pot. Cover the pot and roast for 3½ to 4 hours, until the meat is very soft but not falling apart. Remove the pot from the oven and transfer the meat to a cutting board. Place the pot with the onions on top of the stove. Add the vermouth and bring to a boil. Cook over high heat for 5 minutes, then remove from heat. Add salt and freshly ground black pepper to taste. Cut the meat across the grain into thin slices and return to the pot. Cover the pot, heat gently for 10 minutes, until the meat has soaked in some of the juices, and serve.

Serves 8

CTC	Total Carbs	Fiber	Total Fat	Sat Fat	Protein	Calories
8.15	10.19	2.04	11.15	4.09	35.77	317

tournedos au poivre with balsamic syrup

Slices cut from the heart of a beef tenderloin are called tournedos. If your butcher looks at you askance, simply ask for filet mignon.

4   beef tenderloin fillets (5½ ounces each)
2   tablespoons extra-virgin olive oil
2   teaspoons + 3 tablespoons balsamic vinegar

Place the beef in a shallow baking dish. Pour 1½ tablespoons of the oil over the top and drizzle with 2 teaspoons of the vinegar. Marinate for 1 hour at room temperature, turning frequently.

Remove the fillets from the dish. Sprinkle with salt on both sides. On one side of each fillet, press 2 teaspoons very coarsely ground black pepper.

Lightly coat a cast-iron grill pan or large nonstick skillet with the remaining ½ tablespoon oil. Heat the pan until very hot and cook the fillets for 3 to 4 minutes per side for medium-rare.

Meanwhile, in a small skillet, cook the remaining 3 tablespoons vinegar over high heat until it is reduced to 2 tablespoons.

Transfer the fillets to warm plates. Drizzle each with the reduced balsamic vinegar and a sprinkling of coarse salt and serve immediately.

Serves 4

CTC	Total Carbs	Fiber	Total Fat	Sat Fat	Protein	Calories
1.83	1.83	0	20.16	5.93	32.40	328

pan-seared rib-eye with arugula

There are few things simpler or better than this. It also looks great on the plate. If you find arugula too bitter, you can substitute small, tender leaves of fresh spinach.

4   rib-eye steaks (5½ ounces each)
2   tablespoons garlic-flavored oil
1   large bunch arugula

Place the steaks in a shallow baking dish and drizzle 1 tablespoon of the oil over the top. Sprinkle with coarse salt and freshly ground black pepper. Marinate at room temperature for 1 hour.

Meanwhile, cut the arugula leaves into thin strips, about ¼" wide. Cover and refrigerate until ready to use.

Preheat the oven to 350°F.

Heat a large grill pan or nonstick skillet over high heat until very hot. Add the steaks and cook until charred on the outside and very rare inside, about 2 minutes per side. Transfer the steaks to a rimmed baking sheet and put them in the oven for about 5 minutes, or until they reach the desired doneness, but keeping them as rare as possible for the best results.

Quickly toss the arugula with the remaining 1 tablespoon oil, adding a pinch of salt and pepper. Place a steak in the center of each of 4 large plates and sprinkle lightly with salt. Top each steak with a mound of arugula and serve immediately.

Serves 4

CTC	Total Carbs	Fiber	Total Fat	Sat Fat	Protein	Calories
1.02	1.82	.80	20.02	5.99	32.68	323

singapore steak

There is something remarkable about the way Thai fish sauce alters the color, taste, and texture of an inexpensive cut of meat. Fish sauce, a staple in Southeast Asia, can be found in many supermarkets and any Asian food store. This steak recipe is as delicious as it is unlikely. Serve with an Asian-inspired veggie. Snow Peas with Ginger Butter (page 212), anyone?

4	top round or beef shoulder fillets (7 ounces each)
¼	cup Asian fish sauce
1	bunch scallions

Place the beef in a shallow baking dish. Pour the fish sauce over the beef and turn the beef in the sauce to coat thoroughly.

Set aside 4 of the scallions. Finely mince the remaining scallions to get ¼ cup. Scatter the minced scallions over the steaks. Cover the baking dish and refrigerate for 3 hours, but no longer.

Remove the white parts from the remaining 4 scallions. Make several slits along the length of the white parts, being careful not to cut all the way through. Place the slit scallions in a small bowl of water and put them in the refrigerator. (The scallions will transform themselves into little scallion "brushes" that you will use as a garnish.) Cut the remaining green parts of the scallions on a sharp bias into very thin slices.

When ready to cook, remove the beef from the marinade and pat it dry with paper towels. Heat a large nonstick skillet over high heat until very hot. Sear the beef until charred on the outside and rare on the inside, 3 to 4 minutes per side. Or cook the steaks to the desired doneness.

Transfer the beef to a cutting board. Cut the beef thickly on the bias and place it on 4 warm plates in overlapping slices. Scatter thinly sliced scallion greens on the beef and garnish each with a scallion "brush." Sprinkle the beef with coarse salt and coarsely ground black pepper.

Serves 4

nutritionist's note: With one taste of this, you will never miss the cornstarch-thickened dishes found in typical Asian restaurants that add hidden and unnecessary CTCs.

CTC	Total Carbs	Fiber	Total Fat	Sat Fat	Protein	Calories
4.18	4.83	.65	11.22	4.10	46.94	318

bistecca fiorentina

This is the real thing—Tuscany's low-carb gift to the world of carnivores. You need to use really good olive oil and coarse salt, preferably sea salt. If you're not in a rosemary frame of mind, squeeze fresh lemon juice over the steak instead.

1	porterhouse steak, 1½"-thick (about 1¾ pounds), with bone
¼	cup extra-virgin olive oil
1	bunch fresh rosemary

Place the steak in a large baking dish. Pour 2 tablespoons of the oil over the steak and turn it to coat. Crush about 2 tablespoons of the rosemary leaves and sprinkle them over the steak. Chop the rest of the rosemary and reserve. Crack 1 tablespoon black peppercorns and scatter on top. Let the steak sit at room temperature for 2 hours or longer in the refrigerator.

Preheat the grill until very hot.

Place the steak on the hottest part and grill until still very rare, 5 to 6 minutes per side. Transfer the steak to a cooler area of the grill and continue to cook to the desired doneness.

Transfer the steak to a cutting board. Cut the meat from the bone, then slice the meat on a slight bias into ½"-thick slices. Drizzle the remaining 2 tablespoons oil and any accumulated juices from the board on top of the meat. Sprinkle with coarse salt and cracked black pepper. Garnish with the reserved chopped rosemary. Serve slices from both sides of the bone to each guest, so that everyone gets some of the fillet and some of the sirloin.

Serves 4

CTC	Total Carbs	Fiber	Total Fat	Sat Fat	Protein	Calories
.08	.26	.18	23.27	5.59	38.74	374

chateaubriand with herbes de provence

Present this on a large platter because it is very showy and because, while you parade about the room, the meat can rest and the juices can be reabsorbed. Scented with fragrant herbes de Provence (see page 12), and truffle oil, which is a tad expensive, this is a dish for serving to your favorite guests. You will also need coarse French sea salt (not kosher salt) for this dish if you want to make the truffle roasted salt.

2¾   pounds trimmed fillet of beef, tied with kitchen string in 1½" intervals

2   tablespoons white truffle oil

⅓   cup (or more) herbes de Provence

Preheat the oven to 400°F.

Coat the beef with 1 tablespoon of the truffle oil, using your hands to ensure the entire surface is covered. Sprinkle with salt and grind black pepper all over the beef. Pat the herbes de Provence all over the beef to coat thoroughly, adding more if necessary. Place the beef in the center of a heavy, shallow roasting pan.

Roast the beef for 35 minutes, or until the temperature on an instant-read thermometer reaches between 125° and 130°F for rare, or cook longer if you prefer medium-rare. Transfer the beef to a cutting board and cover it with a foil tent. Let the beef rest for 10 minutes.

Meanwhile, mix 2 tablespoons coarse French sea salt with ½ teaspoon of the remaining truffle oil. Add to a small nonstick skillet and toast over medium heat, stirring constantly, until the salt begins to brown, about 2 minutes. Transfer the salt to a paper towel to cool.

Carve the beef in ½"-thick slices. Drizzle each slice with a little of the remaining 2½ teaspoons truffle oil and serve little mounds of truffle-roasted salt on the side.

Serves 6

CTC	Total Carbs	Fiber	Total Fat	Sat Fat	Protein	Calories
0	.60	.60	19.16	5.81	35.35	326

newspaper-wrapped fillet of beef

New York catering maven Janeen Sarlin discovered that if you wrap a cooked fillet of beef in numerous layers of newspaper, it will stay warm for the better part of the day—and probably taste better for it. An herbal-garlic rub perfumes the meat.

1   whole fillet of beef (5½ pounds), trimmed of fat and tendons and tied
    with kitchen string
1   bulb garlic
1   bunch fresh thyme or rosemary

Let the beef sit at room temperature for 30 minutes.

Preheat the oven to 500°F.

Finely mince the garlic and place it in a bowl. Finely mince the thyme or rosemary to get 2 tablespoons and mix together with the garlic. Add 1 tablespoon coarse salt and 1 tablespoon freshly ground black pepper and mix. Rub this mixture all over the beef.

Place the beef in a rimmed baking sheet or shallow roasting pan. Set the pan in the center of the oven and immediately reduce the heat to 450°F. Roast for 30 minutes, but no longer.

Remove the fillet and wrap it snugly in a sheet of parchment paper. Stack 10 sheets of newspaper on the counter and place the parchment-wrapped fillet on top of the pile of newspapers. Wrap all layers of the newspaper around the fillet, tucking it tightly underneath. Let it sit for at least 30 minutes or up to 2 hours. (Whenever you decide to unwrap the beef, it will still be warm and perfectly done.) Salt the outside of the meat, slice as desired, and serve.

Serves 12

CTC	Total Carbs	Fiber	Total Fat	Sat Fat	Protein	Calories
.81	.92	.11	16.27	6.00	39.45	318

bay leaf-and-beef brochettes

I've never been to the island of Madeira, but I read about this simple recipe in Saveur magazine and immediately co-opted it for a great no-carb outdoor meal. It is known as espetada and was once made by skewering the meat on laurel branches. Long metal skewers will do. Generally it is served with a kind of crumpetlike bread—but you can serve it with a favorite low-carb vegetable. Sautéed Grape Tomatoes with Shallots would do the trick (page 218).

1¾   pounds top sirloin, in 1 piece
6   large cloves garlic
8   bay leaves, fresh if possible, torn into pieces

Trim all but a thin layer of fat from the beef and cut it into 2" cubes.

In a large bowl, combine the beef and 3 tablespoons coarse sea salt. Crush the garlic cloves and add them to the bowl along with the bay leaves. Add lots of freshly ground black pepper, toss to combine, and let sit at room temperature for 1 hour or cover and refrigerate for up to 24 hours for maximum flavor.

Skewer equal amounts of the meat on each of 4 very long metal skewers, beginning and ending with a bay leaf. Grill over a medium-hot grill, turning the skewers often, until browned on all sides, 10 to 12 minutes. Serve immediately.

Serves 4

CTC	Total Carbs	Fiber	Total Fat	Sat Fat	Protein	Calories
.69	.74	.05	15.42	5.84	40.89	313

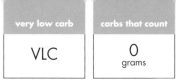
veal loin chops with butter and sage

Veal tends to be delicate, so go easy on the sage. Its flavor will be infused into the brown butter. The 8-ounce veal chops will yield 6½ ounces of meat per serving, before cooking. This tastes rich yet is very low in calories and virtually carb-less.

4   veal loin chops (8 ounces each), ¾" thick
2   tablespoons unsalted butter
1   large bunch fresh sage

Season the veal with salt and freshly ground black pepper. In a nonstick skillet large enough to hold the veal in 1 layer, heat the butter over high heat until it becomes golden brown. Add the veal and cook until browned on the bottom, about 4 minutes. Place 3 sage leaves on the uncooked side of each chop and turn the chops over. Cook until browned on the other side, 3 to 4 minutes longer. Lightly season the veal with salt and coarsely ground black pepper, garnish with a few sage leaves, and serve.

Serves 4

CTC	Total Carbs	Fiber	Total Fat	Sat Fat	Protein	Calories
.04	.11	.07	13.58	6.12	36.88	288

broiled veal steak with fresh thyme mustard

Veal doesn't generally come in "steaks," but I've used inexpensive veal shoulder chops to simulate the steak experience. In addition to broiling, these steaks can easily be made on an outdoor grill.

6	tablespoons Dijon mustard
1	bunch fresh thyme
4	veal shoulder chops (8 ounces each), about ½" thick

Several hours before you plan to serve, place the mustard in a small bowl. Set aside 4 large sprigs of the thyme to use as a garnish and chop the remaining thyme leaves to get 2 tablespoons and stir into the mustard.

Lightly season the veal with salt. Slather all but 2 tablespoons mustard all over the veal chops. Dust with coarsely ground black pepper. Cover and refrigerate 4 to 6 hours.

Preheat the broiler.

Put the veal on a rimmed baking sheet. Broil the veal on 1 side for 3 minutes, until dark golden brown, turn it over, and cook for 2 minutes longer, or until it reaches the desired doneness. (Be careful not to overcook.) Serve the veal immediately with the remaining mustard and garnish with the reserved sprigs of thyme.

Serves 4

CTC	Total Carbs	Fiber	Total Fat	Sat Fat	Protein	Calories
2.00	2.40	.40	9.93	3.02	40.20	276

poultry

Poultry in all forms is the darling of dieters because it contains relatively little fat, particularly if you remove the skin. On the other hand, because today's birds can be bland, they challenge home cooks to produce something tasty, and we're always searching for new recipes to excite our palates.

If only carbs counted, a simple chicken roasted French bistro–style would do. You could rub it with herbs and lots of butter, stick it in the oven till brown and crisp, and serve it forth in all its fatty glory. But this book is as much about calories and health as it is about carbs and waistlines, so we've concentrated on taste while being keenly mindful of the big picture.

Fortunately, there's such an enormous world of flavors to layer onto poultry that there's no danger of ever getting bored. In the recipes that follow, the ingredients keep your palate thoroughly amused: red curry and coconut, salami and roasted peppers, miso and ginger, clove and orange, basil and goat cheese, lemon and chorizo—all sending your taste buds around the world.

A thought about skin: In many cases, I suggest cooking poultry skin-on and then removing the skin before serving. You might well ask why I didn't just start with a skinless bird. There are definite reasons. Skin-on cooking shields a bird's flesh from drying heat and bastes the flesh with flavor. What's more, if you dearly love the crunch of crisp skin and aren't worried about a bit more fat than recommended, you always can "cheat." Keep in mind that you can eat the skin without adding any carbs; you will, however, be adding many calories and a lot of saturated fat. The analyses are calculated, except where noted, without the skin.

When it comes to purchasing chicken, there are many premium brands available today, many claiming to have more flavor. Some are kosher (and are twice-brined), others are free-range, and still others are organic. Also be on the lookout for air-chilled chickens. (Whereas most commercially available chickens are chilled in baths of cold water—some of which they absorb, diluting their flavor—chilling chickens with blasts of frigid air leaves them with more flavor and firmer texture.

Air-chilled chickens are increasingly available in supermarkets, albeit at higher prices than conventional birds.) It might require some experimentation to find the type and brand you like best. Some of my favorites include Murray's Chickens (from the East Coast), D'Artagnan organic chickens (also from the East Coast), and plump Giannone air-chilled chickens from Canada. I suggest you try a basic chicken preparation, like Perfect Chicken Salad (page 151), with a few different brands to determine the one that you like best. After all, this is the time you want your food to taste like . . . well, chicken.

tandoori cornish hens

Indian flavors are speedily being adopted by American chefs, but more slowly at home because of the cuisine's complexity. That's why I recommend a new staple for your pantry: tandoori paste in a jar. These days you can find it in most better supermarkets in the international aisle. It is an aromatic amalgam of ginger, garlic, and other hot and fragrant spices, delicious with shrimp, such as Bombay Shrimp (page 61), or mixed with butter as a topping for grilled meats.

4   Cornish hens (1 pound each)
½   cup tandoori paste
3   cups low-fat plain yogurt

The day before you plan to serve this dish, discard the giblets from the hens or save them for another use. With a sharp knife, make a slash down the center of each hen's breast half and down each leg. Rub about 1 tablespoon of the tandoori paste into the slashes and all over the front and back of each hen. Place the hens in a very large bowl and spread 2 cups of the yogurt over the hens. Toss to completely coat the hens in yogurt. Cover and refrigerate for 12 to 24 hours.

In a small bowl, mix together the remaining 1 cup yogurt with 1 tablespoon of the remaining tandoori paste and a large pinch of salt. Refrigerate until ready to use.

When you are ready to cook the hens, preheat the oven to 400°F.

Scrape off and discard all the marinade from the hens and pat the hens dry with paper towels. Rub each hen with a thin layer of the remaining tandoori paste to cover completely. Place the hens on 2 rimmed baking sheets and bake for 25 minutes. Remove the hens from the oven and baste them with the pan juices.

Preheat the broiler. Remove the tandoori-yogurt sauce from the refrigerator to let it return to room temperature.

Place the hens under the broiler, about 6" from the heat, for about 2 minutes or longer, until blackened in many spots. Remove the hens from the broiler. Remove the skin from the hens. Transfer the hens to a serving platter, pour any pan juices over the hens, and sprinkle them with salt. Serve with the reserved tandoori-yogurt sauce.

Serves 4

CTC	Total Carbs	Fiber	Total Fat	Sat Fat	Protein	Calories
5.34	5.83	.49	9.60	2.71	54.40	340

five-spice roasted chicken

The technique behind this simple dish was inspired by Judy Rodgers, the chef at Zuni Café in San Francisco. The idea is to lightly salt and sugar the bird and leave it uncovered in the refrigerator for a few days before roasting it. The result is very succulent flesh. In this recipe, I've used sugar substitute instead of the sugar, which works perfectly in this capacity.

1	teaspoon granulated sugar substitute
2	tablespoons five-spice powder (see page 12)
1	chicken (4 pounds)

At least 2 days before you plan to serve, in a small bowl, mix together the sugar substitute, five-spice powder, and 2 teaspoons salt. Wash the chicken inside and out and pat it dry with paper towels. Remove and discard the giblets and liver. Remove any extra lobes of fat near the opening of the cavity. Rub the spice mixture all over the surface of the chicken.

Next, dry the skin by placing the chicken on a small wire rack set above a dish and putting it on the top shelf in the refrigerator, uncovered, for 48 hours.

When ready to cook, preheat the oven to 475°F.

Place the chicken, breast side down, in a small roasting pan. Roast for 20 minutes. Turn the chicken over and cook for 20 minutes longer. Reduce the heat to 400°F and cook 20 to 30 minutes longer, or until the temperature on an instant-read thermometer inserted in the thigh reaches 160°F.

Transfer the chicken to a cutting board and let it rest for 10 minutes. Add 1 cup boiling water to the juices in the pan and cook for 1 minute over high heat, scraping up any bits. Pour the juices through a fine-mesh strainer into a small saucepan. Bring the juices to a boil, add salt and freshly ground black pepper to taste, and remove from the heat. Carve the chicken as desired. Remove the skin and serve immediately with warm juices.

Serves 4

nutritionist's note: When a recipe calls for a whole chicken, the analysis per serving includes some white and dark meat. If you choose just white meat (breast), each ounce has 31 calories, almost no saturated fat, and 0 CTC. Dark meat has 34 calories per ounce, about .5 gram saturated fat, and 0 CTC.

CTC	Total Carbs	Fiber	Total Fat	Sat Fat	Protein	Calories
.99	2.84	1.85	5.54	1.43	56.12	298

poulet aux champignons

This is the classic French method for roasting chicken: massaging it with butter before cooking and finishing the sauce with a bit of butter to make it silky. Dried mushrooms make a robust stock and flavor.

1	cup dried porcini or shiitake mushrooms
1	chicken (5 pounds)
4	tablespoons unsalted butter

Preheat the oven to 375°F.

Place the mushrooms in a bowl and pour 2 cups boiling water over them. Soak the mushrooms for 20 minutes. Over a bowl, pour the mushrooms and soaking liquid into a fine-mesh strainer. Transfer the mushrooms to a separate bowl. Reserve the soaking liquid.

Wash the chicken inside and out and pat it dry with paper towels. Reserve the giblets and discard the liver. Remove any lobes of fat near the opening of the cavity. Season the chicken inside and out with salt and freshly ground black pepper.

In a small skillet over medium heat, melt 1 tablespoon of the butter. Add the mushrooms and cook, stirring, for 5 minutes. Fill the cavity of the chicken with the mushrooms and truss the bird. Use your fingers to spread 1 tablespoon of the butter on the chicken breast. Place the chicken in a heavy, shallow roasting pan and roast for about 90 minutes, or until the temperature on an instant-read thermometer inserted in the thigh reaches 160°F. Meanwhile, put the giblets in a small saucepan with ½ cup water and the reserved mushroom liquid. Bring the liquid to a boil, then reduce the heat and simmer for 25 minutes. Discard the giblets. Pour the liquid through a strainer into a medium saucepan.

Transfer the chicken to a cutting board with a well. Tilt the chicken to collect the juices and add them to the mushroom liquid. Scoop the mushrooms out of the chicken cavity and add to the mushroom liquid. Add ½ cup boiling water to the roasting pan and cook for 1 minute over high heat, scraping up any browned bits. Strain the pan juices into the mushroom liquid. Cook over high heat until reduced by two-thirds. Add 2 tablespoons butter and whisk constantly until the sauce emulsifies, about 1 minute. Add salt and pepper to taste. Carve the chicken and remove the skin. Serve with warm sauce.

Serves 6

nutritionist's note: Surprisingly, dried mushrooms are a good source of fiber. This analysis is based on some white and dark meat. For all white meat, the calories and saturated fat will be a bit lower.

CTC	Total Carbs	Fiber	Total Fat	Sat Fat	Protein	Calories
1.89	6.61	4.72	12.76	6.07	51.70	362

david feder's tahini chicken

David Feder, a former Middle Eastern archaeologist and food editor at Better Homes & Gardens *for years, is also an exceptional chef. He makes this Levantine-inspired dish every Friday night for his family. Be certain to use pure tahini, which you can get at Middle Eastern and health food stores.*

3	tablespoons fennel seeds
¼	cup tahini (sesame seed paste)
1	chicken (3½ pounds)

Preheat the oven to 375°F.

In a spice mill or coffee grinder, pulverize the fennel seeds until they are coarsely ground.

In a small bowl, mix together the fennel seeds, 2 teaspoons salt, and a liberal grinding of black pepper.

Stir the tahini in the jar, making sure to incorporate any oil that may have risen to the top. Scoop ¼ cup tahini into a bowl along with half of the fennel mixture. Stir to incorporate.

Wash the chicken inside and out and pat it dry with paper towels. Discard the giblets and liver or save them for another use. Gently loosen the chicken skin from the flesh, taking care not to tear the skin. (You'll find specific instructions for this in my recipe for Basil-and-Chèvre-Stuffed Chicken on the opposite page.) Lean the chicken on something to hold it upright. Spoon half of the tahini mixture under the skin over each breast. Then use your finger to spread the tahini paste over the flesh under the skin of the chicken and onto the drumsticks and thighs. Rub the outside of the chicken with the remaining fennel mixture.

Place the chicken, breast side up, on a roasting rack in a foil-lined roasting pan. Roast for 1 hour and 15 minutes, or until the chicken is golden brown, the drumsticks can be moved freely, and the juices run clear when the tip of a small knife is inserted in the thigh.

Remove the chicken from the oven and let it stand for 10 minutes before carving. Remove the skin before serving.

Serves 4

nutritionist's note: The analysis for each serving is based on some white and dark meat. Calories and saturated fat will be slightly lower for all white meat.

CTC	Total Carbs	Fiber	Total Fat	Sat Fat	Protein	Calories
3.88	5.88	2.00	12.23	2.23	45.87	323

basil-and-chèvre-stuffed chicken

This is a show-off dish that results in an extraordinarily plump bird. Forcing the basil-speckled cheese mixture under the skin takes a bit of patience, but it infuses the flesh with enormous flavor and keeps it ultra juicy. Use a good-quality fresh goat cheese such as one from France or a great domestic variety such as Coach Farms.

1	chicken (5 pounds)
2	large bunches fresh basil
6	ounces fresh goat cheese (chèvre)

Preheat the oven to 375°F.

Remove the giblets and liver from the chicken and discard or save them for another use. Remove any lobes of fat near the opening of the cavity. Wash the chicken inside and out and pat it dry with paper towels.

Pick off 3 packed cups of basil leaves. In a food processor, combine the basil and goat cheese. Add a pinch of salt and a generous amount of coarsely ground black pepper. Process until the cheese is smooth, being careful not to overprocess.

Now insert the cheese under the chicken's skin: Starting at the neck, slip your fingers under the breast skin, carefully separating the skin from the flesh. Moving your fingers left and right, continue downward and, with your index finger, separate the skin around the thighs. The chicken's skin is flexible enough so that it won't tear, even as you probe toward the thighs. With your fingers or a spoon, push the cheese mixture under the skin to cover the entire breast and thighs, using all of the mixture. You will have approximately a ¼" layer of cheese under the skin. Press on the skin to evenly distribute the cheese.

Truss the chicken. Sprinkle the chicken lightly with salt and freshly ground black pepper. Place the chicken in a heavy shallow, roasting pan and roast for 1½ hours, or until the temperature on an instant-read thermometer inserted in the thigh reaches 160°F. Remove the chicken from the oven and let it rest for 10 minutes before carving. Remove the skin before serving.

Serves 6

nutritionist's note: I suggest not eating the skin because it will put the saturated fat way over the top and, of course, add calories. However, it will not add any carbs, so the choice is up to you.

CTC	Total Carbs	Fiber	Total Fat	Sat Fat	Protein	Calories
.34	1.17	.83	11.53	5.54	55.60	344

salt-baked rosemary chicken

Parade this chicken around the dining room table before dramatically cracking open its salt crust and releasing the enticing aromas. The moist, herb-infused meat gets anointed with peppery lemon oil. Note: You will need about 4 pounds of kosher salt for this recipe.

1   chicken (4 pounds)
2   large bunches fresh rosemary
3   tablespoons + 1 teaspoon lemon-flavored olive oil

Preheat the oven to 450°F.

Pour 2 cups kosher salt into the bottom of a deep ovenproof baking dish with a cover.

Remove the giblets and liver from the chicken and discard or save them for another use. Wash the chicken inside and out and pat it dry with paper towels. Fill the cavity with rosemary, saving some to use as a garnish.

Put the chicken on top of the salt, breast side up. Add salt to cover the top and sides of the chicken, about 8 cups more. Sprinkle with 1 cup water, patting down the salt to make a solid crust. Bake, covered, for 45 minutes. Remove the cover and bake for 20 minutes more. Remove the baking dish from the oven and let the chicken rest for 10 minutes.

Meanwhile, in a small bowl, mix together the oil, a pinch of salt, and ½ teaspoon coarsely ground black pepper. Set aside.

Display the chicken to your family or guests, then crack the salt crust with the back of a heavy knife. Remove the chicken from the salt. Remove all the salt with a pastry brush. Remove the skin and carve the chicken as desired. Serve with the lemon-pepper oil for drizzling over the chicken and garnish with rosemary sprigs.

Serves 4

nutritionist's note: Heart-healthy olive oil is carb free, so you may drizzle more over your portion. However, every tablespoon of olive oil has 120 calories.

CTC	Total Carbs	Fiber	Total Fat	Sat Fat	Protein	Calories
.07	.15	.08	18.31	3.24	55.53	398

za'atar chicken

Za'atar is a heady, khaki-colored spice mixture that includes dried hyssop (rather like wild thyme or marjoram), sumac, and sesame seeds, imparting a robust flavor profile to this plain old chicken. Generally used in Lebanon, Jordan, and Israel, you should be able to find this spice mix in any Middle Eastern food shop.

8   medium to large chicken thighs (about 3¼ pounds), bone-in
⅔   cup za'atar
3   lemons

Remove the skin from the chicken thighs and discard. Place the chicken in a shallow baking dish and rub it well with ½ cup of the za'atar. Grate the zest of 2 lemons and sprinkle it over the chicken. Cut the lemons in half and squeeze the juice over the chicken. Add freshly ground black pepper and roll the chicken around in the mixture. Cover the chicken and refrigerate for 3 to 4 hours.

Preheat the oven to 375°F.

Place the chicken on a heavy baking sheet or in a shallow broiler pan. Bake for 45 minutes. Transfer the chicken to a warm platter and cover with foil. Add 1 cup boiling water to the baking sheet and scrape up the pan juices. Transfer the juices to a small saucepan and boil until the sauce is thickened, about 1 minute. Pour over the chicken and sprinkle with the remaining za'atar. Top with thin slices of the remaining lemon.

Serves 4

CTC	Total Carbs	Fiber	Total Fat	Sat Fat	Protein	Calories
6.23	10.54	4.31	11.78	2.50	48.50	352

chicken breasts with slow-roasted grapes

Roasted grapes provide concentrated, intense bursts of sweet-tart flavor, and the acidity in reduced fresh grape juice emulsifies the butter into a rich, sweet, mahogany-colored sauce.

1	pound seedless dark red grapes
3	tablespoons unsalted butter
4	skinless, boneless chicken breasts (6 ounces each)

Preheat the oven to 275°F.

Remove the grapes from their stems. Place half of the grapes on a rimmed baking sheet. Bake for 1½ hours, shaking the pan frequently. Remove from the oven and set aside.

Place the uncooked grapes in a blender and puree until very smooth. Strain through a coarse-mesh sieve into a bowl, pressing down hard on the skins. Discard the skins and set aside the juice.

In a large nonstick skillet over medium-high heat, melt 2 tablespoons of the butter. Season the chicken with salt and freshly ground black pepper. Add the chicken to the skillet and cook until golden, about 5 minutes per side.

Add the grape juice and cook until the chicken is done and just firm to the touch, about 5 minutes longer. (Be careful not to overcook.) The grape juices will darken into a mahogany-colored sauce. Transfer the chicken to a platter.

Add the remaining 1 tablespoon butter to the skillet and cook over high heat, stirring, for 1 minute. Add the oven-dried grapes and cook, stirring, for 1 minute longer. Add salt and pepper to taste and pour the sauce over the chicken. Serve immediately.

Serves 4

nutritionist's note: This dish is worth the indulgent level of CTC. The roasted red grapes provide flavonoids—compounds that can help prevent heart disease—and add natural sweetness to the suave sauce.

CTC	Total Carbs	Fiber	Total Fat	Sat Fat	Protein	Calories
18.32	19.45	1.13	11.14	6.07	40.08	339

asian chicken with scallions

This may become your family's favorite dish. It is slightly mysterious because the chicken marinates in Asian fish sauce (known as nam pla *and* nuoc nam*), a staple of many dishes in southeast Asia. You can find it in many supermarkets and certainly in Asian food stores. This is a great dish for a picnic, served at room temperature or chilled.*

4	large chicken breast halves on the bone (about 10 ounces each), with skin
¼	cup Asian fish sauce
4	scallions

The day before you plan to serve, cut each chicken breast in half across the width of the breast. Place the chicken in a bowl and pour the fish sauce over. Toss to coat thoroughly.

Remove 3" of the dark green part of the scallions and discard. Cut each of the scallions very thin, on the bias, about ⅛" thick. Add the scallions to the bowl with the chicken and toss. Cover and refrigerate for 18 to 24 hours.

Preheat the oven to 500°F.

Lift the chicken from the fish sauce, letting the scallion slices remain on the chicken. Place the chicken on a rimmed baking sheet. Bake for 10 to 12 minutes, until just firm, then put under the broiler, about 8" from the heat, for 1 to 2 minutes, until just golden. Remove from the oven. Remove the skin and serve immediately, if serving hot. Or you can serve the chicken at room temperature or chilled.

Serves 4

nutritionist's note: The secret to success with this dish is not to tell your family what's in it. Fish sauce, made from fermented anchovies, would have been a turn-off to my kids, but now they ask for this low-carb (and low sat fat) chicken dish all the time!

CTC	Total Carbs	Fiber	Total Fat	Sat Fat	Protein	Calories
3.56	4.21	.65	3.57	.94	67.49	336

chicken rollatini with salami and roasted peppers

These roll-ups take chicken in an Italian direction, with both salami and roasted peppers keeping the breasts moist. I like the purity of freshly roasted peppers, but jarred ones are just fine; in fact, they add an appealing touch of vinegar to the chicken. Ask your butcher to remove the bones from the chicken breasts, or you can easily do it yourself using a small, sharp knife.

2   jarred roasted red peppers
4   large chicken breast halves on the bone (about 10 ounces each), with skin
4   ounces preservative-free organic salami, thinly sliced

Preheat the oven to 350°F.

Cut the roasted peppers into ½"-wide by 3"-long strips and set aside.

Remove the bones and the "tenders" from the breasts and set aside. (Tenders are the small muscles running the length of the breasts, approximately ½" in diameter, under each breast half.) Place the breasts on a flat surface, skin side down. Flatten the breasts slightly with a cleaver or mallet and season with salt and freshly ground black pepper.

Place an overlapping layer of the salami on a chicken breast to cover the flesh. Place several strips of red pepper down the center of the breast. Place a chicken tender on top of the pepper. Tightly roll up the chicken breasts, jelly-roll style, to completely envelop the filling. Repeat with the remaining chicken breasts.

Season the rollatinis with salt and pepper and place them on a rimmed baking sheet. Bake for 25 minutes. Place under the broiler, about 6" from the heat, for about 30 seconds to crisp the skin.

Remove the rollatinis from the oven and let rest for 5 minutes. Cut each rollatini on a slight bias into 5 thick slices. Remove the skin. Serve overlapping slices with pan juices drizzled on top.

Serves 4

nutritionist's note: The skin helps hold the chicken rollatini together and keeps the juices from running away. When its job is done, you can remove the skin because this dish is great enough without the extra fat and calories. Again, the choice is up to you; the skin adds no carbs.

CTC	Total Carbs	Fiber	Total Fat	Sat Fat	Protein	Calories
2.98	4.17	1.19	12.01	4.08	52.22	344

lemon chicken and chorizo

The lemon in this recipe serves two purposes. It perks up flavor, and it binds all the juices in this one-pan dish into a robust sauce. Chorizos are hard sausages with Mexican or Spanish overtones. Some are smokey, and others are highly piquant. Pepperoni makes an acceptable substitute. Preservative-free organic chorizo and pepperoni have become readily available. Although a bit pricier, I think it is worth the extra money to avoid the nitrites present in standard products.

4   ounces chorizo sausage
8   medium chicken thighs (about 3 pounds), bone-in
3   large lemons

Slice the chorizo into ¼"-thick rounds and put them into a large nonreactive bowl. Add the chicken. Grate the zest of the lemons and add to the bowl with ½ teaspoon coarse salt and freshly ground black pepper. Toss all of the ingredients together and refrigerate for 4 to 6 hours.

With a sharp knife, cut the rind and pith from the lemons. Cut the lemon flesh into ¼" dice, removing any seeds. Set aside.

Heat a large nonstick skillet over medium-high heat. Place the chicken, skin side down, in the skillet along with the chorizo. Cook until the chicken is golden, about 10 minutes. Turn the chicken over and cook it until the chicken is cooked through and the chorizo is browned, about 10 minutes longer. Add the diced lemon and increase the heat to high. Cook 3 to 4 minutes more. (The lemon will emulsify and thicken the pan juices.) Remove the skin, season with salt and pepper to taste, and serve.

Serves 4

CTC	Total Carbs	Fiber	Total Fat	Sat Fat	Protein	Calories
5.38	9.19	3.81	19.65	6.29	47.65	393

chipotle chicken

Chipotle chile peppers are what Mexicans call smoked jalapeño peppers. They're available canned in adobo sauce in Mexican and Latino food markets and in the ethnic section of good supermarkets and are both spicy and flavorful. Mixing them with grated onions creates a marinade that permeates the chicken and tenderizes it at the same time. This is great on the grill.

3   medium red onions
4   chipotle chile peppers in adobo sauce
4   large chicken breast halves on the bone (about 10 ounces each), with skin

Grate 1 onion on the large holes of a box grater. Place the grated onion and its juices in a large bowl. Thinly slice the remaining onions and add them to the bowl. Chop the chipotle peppers with a little of their sauce and add to the bowl along with the chicken breasts. Add ½ teaspoon coarse salt and toss well. Cover and refrigerate for 1 hour.

Preheat the oven to 350°F.

On a rimmed baking sheet or in a shallow broiler pan, place the chicken along with its marinade, slipping onion slices under the breasts. Bake for 40 minutes or until the chicken is cooked through. (Do not overcook; you want the chicken to be juicy and moist.) Remove the chicken from the oven and remove the skin. Top the chicken with the browned onions, add salt to taste, and serve.

Serves 4

CTC	Total Carbs	Fiber	Total Fat	Sat Fat	Protein	Calories
6.85	8.91	2.06	3.15	.79	53.53	290

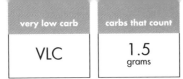

very low carb	carbs that count
VLC	1.5 grams

pecan-crusted chicken breasts

Replacing the skin of the chicken in this straightforward dish is a layer of pesto and crushed pecans that form a desirable crust, adding texture and helping to seal in the juices. Because of the moist texture and vibrant flavors, it is also delicious served cold.

3   ounces pecans (about ⅔ cup)
4   large chicken breasts halves on the bone (about 1½ pounds total),
    with skin
4   ounces prepared pesto (about ½ cup)

In a food processor, briefly process the pecans until they are coarsely ground.

Preheat the oven to 425°F.

Remove the skin from the chicken and discard. Thickly coat the top of each breast with pesto. Then pack the ground pecans onto the pesto to thoroughly cover.

Place the chicken on a rimmed baking sheet. Sprinkle each breast with salt and freshly ground black pepper. Bake for 30 minutes. Serve immediately with any pan juices drizzled on top.

Serves 4

CTC	Total Carbs	Fiber	Total Fat	Sat Fat	Protein	Calories
1.62	4.75	3.13	22.76	3.17	43.92	399

miso chicken with fresh ginger

This simple chicken dish is amazing because miso, fermented soybean paste, is a great carrier of flavors. Miso can be found in the refrigerated section in health food stores and Asian markets. You can make this dish with fresh ginger or prepare it with garlic cloves pushed through a press. I really can't decide which I like better—so sometimes I make a platter of each for parties. In that case, do chicken breasts with ginger and thighs with garlic. If using garlic, push 4 large cloves through a garlic press and add to the miso-water mixture.

⅓   cup white (shiro) miso
1   6" piece fresh ginger
4   large chicken breast halves on the bone (about 10 ounces each),
    with skin

The day before you plan to serve, in a large bowl, combine the miso and ⅓ cup cold water and whisk until thoroughly combined, smooth, and thick.

Using a small, sharp knife, peel the ginger. Grate the ginger on the large holes of a box grater. Wrap the grated ginger in a paper towel and squeeze the ginger juice, about 2 tablespoons, through the paper towel into the bowl with the miso. Stir to incorporate.

Cut the chicken breasts in half across the width of each breast. Add the chicken to the miso-ginger mixture and turn the pieces to coat thoroughly. Sprinkle the chicken liberally with salt. For a more gingery flavor, you can finely chop the remaining ginger pulp, add it to the chicken, and mix again. Cover and refrigerate for 18 to 24 hours.

Preheat the oven to 500°F.

Remove the chicken from the bowl, making sure some marinade remains on the chicken, and transfer to a rimmed baking sheet, skin side up. Bake for 10 minutes, then put under the broiler, about 6" from the heat, for 1 to 2 minutes, or until the skin is dark golden brown and the chicken is just firm to the touch. (Be careful not to overcook.) Remove the skin and serve immediately.

Serves 4

CTC	Total Carbs	Fiber	Total Fat	Sat Fat	Protein	Calories
6.10	7.48	1.38	4.96	1.15	68.29	364

red curry-coconut chicken breasts

You can catch the wave of incendiary Thai cuisine with a quick trip to your supermarket's Asian food section, where you'll probably find two of the ingredients required for this recipe. The red curry paste has lots of heat, which is tempered into a creamy sauce by the light coconut milk.

4   large chicken breast halves on the bone (about 10 ounces each), with skin

2   tablespoons red curry paste

1⅓ cups light coconut milk

Up to 1 day before you plan to serve, using a sharp knife, make 3 deep slashes across the width of each chicken breast. Rub ½ tablespoon curry paste into the flesh of each breast, making sure some of the paste gets into the slits. Place the chicken in a shallow baking dish and pour ⅓ cup of the coconut milk over each breast. Sprinkle liberally with salt. Cover the baking dish and refrigerate for 8 to 24 hours.

Preheat the oven to 475°F.

Remove the chicken from the marinade, reserving the marinade separately, and place the chicken on a rimmed baking sheet. Bake for 25 minutes or until the chicken is firm to the touch. (Do not overcook.)

Meanwhile, in a small saucepan, bring the reserved marinade to a boil. Let it boil for 1 to 2 minutes, lower the heat to medium, and cook for 5 minutes longer. Remove from the heat and add salt to taste.

Remove the chicken from the oven, transfer it to a platter, and sprinkle it lightly with salt. Spoon the hot sauce over the chicken and serve immediately.

Serves 4

nutritionist's note: By using light coconut milk instead of regular, you save 8 grams of saturated fat and still have great coconut flavor.

CTC	Total Carbs	Fiber	Total Fat	Sat Fat	Protein	Calories
2.99	2.99	0	8.30	5.24	53.37	312

quick chicken parmigiana

Chicken "parm" is one of America's most popular dishes, but it always comes breaded and fried. I've low-carbed it here (and slashed the calories) by scrapping the breading but not its essential Italian spirit, nor the oozing melted cheese. This is perfect for a get-it-on-the-table-fast lunch or supper.

4   skinless, boneless chicken breasts (8 ounces each)
1   cup marinara sauce
3½ ounces provolone cheese, thinly sliced

In a large, deep, nonstick sauté pan, add salted water to a depth of 2" and bring to a boil. Slip the chicken into the water and reduce the heat to medium. Cook until the chicken is just firm to the touch, about 10 minutes. Immediately remove the chicken from the water and pat it dry with paper towels. Season the chicken with salt and ground white pepper.

Preheat the broiler.

Spray a rimmed baking sheet with cooking spray.

In a small nonstick skillet over medium heat, add the sauce and heat until just hot.

Place the still-warm chicken on the baking sheet. Spoon the sauce evenly over the chicken and cover them with the cheese. Broil about 6" from the heat until the cheese is a little bubbly and golden brown. Remove the chicken from the oven and serve immediately.

Serves 4

nutritionist's note: Many jarred marinara sauces are very high in added sugars. Check the nutrition labels and buy one that contains no more than 5 grams of carbohydrates per ½ cup.

CTC	Total Carbs	Fiber	Total Fat	Sat Fat	Protein	Calories
5.03	6.53	1.50	12.41	5.73	59.71	392

chicken "al souk"

Some alchemy occurs when you marinate meat or poultry in a mixture of grated onion and yogurt—a technique popular in eastern Mediterranean countries. The flesh becomes remarkably juicy and very tender. Here additional onion is caramelized and strewn atop the finished dish. Yum.

3   medium yellow onions
1   cup low-fat plain yogurt
8   medium to large chicken thighs, with skin

Up to 1 day before you plan to serve, cut 1 onion in half. Grate ½ onion on the large holes of a box grater and transfer the grated onion and its juices to a large bowl. Set aside the other onion half. Dice a second onion into ⅛" pieces and add them to the bowl. (You will have about 2 cups.) Add the yogurt, ½ teaspoon salt, and lots of freshly ground black pepper and mix well.

With a sharp knife, remove skin and lobes of fat from the thighs and reserve. Toss the chicken in the onion-yogurt mixture to coat completely. Cover and refrigerate for 8 to 12 hours.

Preheat the oven to 350°F.

Place the chicken on a rimmed baking sheet, making sure that the pieces are not crowded and are well covered with yogurt and onions. Bake for 45 minutes, then set under the broiler, about 6" from the heat. Broil until the onions are somewhat blackened, about 4 minutes.

Meanwhile, in a medium nonstick skillet over medium-high heat, add the reserved fat and skin and heat until 1 tablespoon fat is rendered. Remove the skin and any solid fat, leaving the rendered fat in the skillet. Slice the remaining 1½ onions half paper-thin and add to the hot chicken fat. Cook over high heat, stirring often, until the onion turns dark brown, about 5 minutes.

Remove the chicken from the oven and spoon any pan juices over the chicken. Sprinkle with salt and top with the sautéed onions.

Serves 4

nutritionist's note: Here, chicken fat (1 tablespoon rendered from the chicken skin) is used to cook the onions. Chicken fat has about half the saturated fat and almost twice the good monounsaturated fat of butter.

CTC	Total Carbs	Fiber	Total Fat	Sat Fat	Protein	Calories
10.13	11.62	1.49	11.96	3.46	42.95	334

warm poached chicken with sun-dried tomatoes and capers

The unusual and ever so simple cooking method—borrowed from the Chinese—yields meltingly tender flesh. Juices from the sun-dried tomatoes and capers coalesce into a warm vinaigrette. This is a perfect dish for a special lunch, requiring very little effort.

1	whole chicken (4 pounds)
¾	cup sun-dried tomatoes in olive oil
2–3	tablespoons capers

Rinse the chicken inside and out. Remove the giblets and liver from the chicken, discard the liver, and put the giblets in a pot large enough to comfortably accommodate the chicken. Truss the chicken and place it in the pot with the giblets. Cover completely with cold water. Add 3 tablespoons kosher salt and 1 tablespoon whole black peppercorns. Cover the pot and bring the water to a rapid boil. This will take 20 to 25 minutes. Do not lift the cover, just listen for the water to boil. Turn off the heat, do not lift the cover, and let it sit for 3½ hours.

While the chicken is cooking, coarsely chop the sun-dried tomatoes and transfer them, with their oil, to a small saucepan. Add the capers, plus a little brine to taste.

Transfer the chicken to a large cutting board. Discard the skin and remove the meat from the bones in large pieces. Arrange the chicken on a warm platter and cover it with foil. Strain the poaching liquid through a fine-mesh sieve and save it for another use, such as making soup. My husband loves to eat the carb-free giblets.

Gently warm the sun-dried tomatoes and capers, adding a few tablespoons of the poaching liquid if desired, then pour over the chicken and serve immediately.

Serves 4

CTC	Total Carbs	Fiber	Total Fat	Sat Fat	Protein	Calories
3.73	5.13	1.40	9.60	2.12	56.70	343

perfect chicken salad

This simple technique, similar to the preceding recipe, yields a memorable texture that is perfect for cold preparations where moisture is key. As a bonus, you can reduce the broth to use as a base for chicken soup. Chop the chicken into small chunks for an open-face sandwich or lettuce wrapper or cut it into long, thin strips as a main-course salad.

1   chicken (3 pounds)
1   cup chopped celery
1   cup light mayonnaise

Rinse the chicken, inside and out, discarding the giblets and liver. Put the chicken in a pot large enough to accommodate it. Cover the chicken with cold water. Add 3 tablespoons kosher salt and bring the water to a rapid boil. Submerge the chicken and bring the water to a boil again, uncovered. Boil for 15 minutes, then turn off the heat, cover, and let the chicken remain in the water for 20 minutes.

Remove the chicken from the water and reserve the broth for another use, such as making soup. Also reserve about ½ cup broth for moistening the chicken salad later on. Let the chicken cool until you can handle it easily. Pull out as many bones as possible and refrigerate the chicken until it is cold. Remove all bones and skin and cut the chicken into small chunks or into long strips.

Place the chicken in a bowl and toss with the celery and mayonnaise. Add a few tablespoons of the reserved broth to moisten the chicken salad, if necessary. Add salt and ground white pepper to taste. Chill again.

Serves 6 (makes about 2 pounds)

CTC	Total Carbs	Fiber	Total Fat	Sat Fat	Protein	Calories
3.06	3.40	.34	17.21	3.67	37.72	332

cold poached chicken with avocado and mango

What do you get when you whip together a juicy ripe mango and a fleshy avocado? A beautiful sauce with intriguing flavor and mousselike texture that tastes great on cold poached chicken. Avocados, once a no-no on many diets, are a source of "good" fat.

4 skinless, boneless chicken breasts (6 ounces each)
1 medium ripe mango
1 medium ripe avocado

In a large, deep, nonstick sauté pan, add 2" of salted water. Bring the water to a boil. Slip the chicken breasts into the sauté pan and cook for 2 minutes, then turn the chicken over and cook for another 2 minutes. Cover the pan, reduce the heat to a simmer, and cook for 2 minutes longer. Remove from the heat and let sit for 5 minutes, covered, or until the chicken is just firm to the touch. Remove the chicken from the water, wrap it in plastic, and refrigerate it until it is cold.

Shortly before serving, using a small, sharp knife, remove the skin from the mango. Cut the flesh away from the pit. Cut ¾ of the mango flesh into chunks and put it in a blender. Cut the avocado in half lengthwise, around the pit. Twist to separate the sides and remove the pit. Scoop out the flesh from 1 avocado half and cut it into chunks. Add the chunks to the blender. Add a pinch of salt and 2 tablespoons water to the blender and process until very smooth. You will have about 1⅓ cups sauce.

Cut the chilled chicken into thick slices on the bias, across the width of the breast. Arrange the chicken in overlapping slices on serving plates. Sprinkle with salt and ground white pepper. Slice the remaining mango quarter and avocado half into thin slices and use them as garnishes. Serve with the sauce spooned over, or under, the chicken. Pass the pepper mill at the table.

Serves 4

CTC	Total Carbs	Fiber	Total Fat	Sat Fat	Protein	Calories
9.07	12.51	3.44	9.95	1.82	40.54	302

golden capon with 40 cloves of garlic

You don't see capon very often these days because ever-larger chickens are ever-more available. A capon is a castrated rooster that has more fat and flesh than a typical chicken and amply serves 6 people. The excess of garlic melts into a sweet sauce augmented by the nutty taste of dry sherry. This is one of my favorite offerings at the holiday table, when I'm serving two main courses.

1   capon (8 pounds)
40   large cloves garlic, peeled
¾   cup dry sherry

Preheat the oven to 400°F.

Rinse the capon inside and out and dry it well with paper towels. Remove the giblets and liver and discard the liver. Put the giblets in a small saucepan with 3 cups of water to cover. Add 1 clove garlic, slightly smashed, and ¼ teaspoon black peppercorns to the saucepan. Bring the water to a boil, then reduce the heat and simmer for 30 minutes. Strain through a sieve into a clean saucepan. Cook the broth over medium heat until it is reduced to 1 cup. Set aside.

Meanwhile, press 2 cloves garlic through a garlic press and rub it all over the capon. Season the capon with salt and freshly ground black pepper. Tie the legs together with kitchen string.

Place the capon breast side up in a shallow roasting pan. Surround the capon with the remaining garlic cloves. Roast the capon for 30 minutes, then reduce the oven temperature to 350°F and roast 1 hour longer, basting often, or until an instant-read thermometer inserted in the thigh reaches a temperature of 160°F and the juices run clear. Transfer the capon and garlic to a cutting board and tent with foil while you prepare the sauce.

Pour all but 1 tablespoon fat from the roasting pan. Place the pan on the stove top over high heat. Add the 1 cup reduced stock and the sherry and scrape up any browned bits in the pan with a spatula. Pour the liquid through a sieve into a clean saucepan and bring it to a boil. Reduce the heat and simmer until the sauce becomes a bit syrupy, about 5 minutes. Carve the capon as desired, drizzle with the sauce, and serve with the garlic cloves.

Serves 6

nutritionist's note: Dry sherry does a great low-carb job of flavoring this sauce. Feel free to sip a little while cooking! Four ounces has less than 1.5 grams of carbohydrates.

CTC	Total Carbs	Fiber	Total Fat	Sat Fat	Protein	Calories
6.56	6.98	.42	7.31	1.97	50.77	339

pot-roasted turkey thigh with smokey onions

I hope you can find very big turkey thighs like I often can in my supermarket, because this is one of my new favorite "cuts" of meat. One large thigh weighs about 1¾ pounds and feeds two beautifully. My method—half roasted/half "potted"—yields the most succulent meat that can be carved into ½"-thick juicy slices. Smoked paprika and onions turn into a smokey, intensely flavored, thick, jammy sauce. You can find smoked paprika, exported from Spain, in gourmet food and spice stores and many upscale supermarkets. It lasts a long time in your pantry and will become one of your favorite spices! This is a great dinner for two. If serving more, use a larger baking dish.

1   medium-large yellow onion
1   very large turkey thigh (about 1¾ pounds)
1   tablespoon smoked paprika

Preheat the oven to 425°F.

You will need a shallow, metal casserole with a cover for the best results. The baking pan should be only a little larger than the thigh. (A Le Creuset enameled cast-iron pan is perfect.) Cut the onion in half through the equator. Slice half of the onion ⅛" thick. Spread the onion slices over the bottom of the baking pan.

Grate the other onion half on the large holes of a box grater. Rub the onion pulp and juices all over the turkey. Sprinkle the turkey with the smoked paprika and lightly with salt. Place the turkey on top of the onions in the baking pan.

Bake the turkey, uncovered, for 20 minutes. Reduce the heat to 325°F. Cover the baking pan tightly and bake 50 to 60 minutes longer, until the turkey is very tender and the onions are darkly caramelized. Halfway through the cooking time, baste the turkey with some of the pan juices.

Remove the turkey from the oven and transfer it to a cutting board. Remove the skin, carve the turkey into ½"-thick slices, and arrange it on 2 large plates. Spoon the cooked onions and pan juices over the turkey and serve immediately.

Serves 2

CTC	Total Carbs	Fiber	Total Fat	Sat Fat	Protein	Calories
4.85	6.50	1.65	6.55	2.12	47.51	282

rolled-and-tied turkey with pears

I love this cut of turkey, which most butchers carry—half of a large turkey breast with the skin on and bones removed. It looks like and can be used as London broil. Here it is rubbed with herbs and tied like a roast. Baked pears transform into a delectable sauce. Substitute fresh sage and this becomes a great autumn dish; lemon balm makes it taste like spring.

1   large bunch fresh basil
1   turkey "London broil," half breast with bones removed (2½ pounds)
3   large ripe Comice pears

Preheat the oven to 400°F.

Chop enough basil to get ½ cup, reserving some whole basil leaves and a few sprigs for garnishing.

Place the turkey on a board, skin side down. Spread the chopped basil on the turkey and season it with salt and freshly ground black pepper. Roll the turkey lengthwise to make a cylindrical shape, about 10" long and 4" wide at the widest point in the center. Tie with kitchen string at 1½" intervals. Again, season the turkey with salt and pepper. Tuck some of the reserved whole basil leaves under the strings to cover the top.

Peel the pears and halve them lengthwise, removing the seeds. Place the turkey in a shallow roasting pan and arrange the pears, cut sides down, around it.

Bake the turkey for 45 to 50 minutes, or until the temperature on an instant-read thermometer inserted into the thickest part reaches 150°F. Transfer the turkey and pears to a cutting board.

Pour ½ cup boiling water into the roasting pan set over medium-high heat on top of the stove and scrape up any browned bits. Pour the pan juices into a blender. Roughly chop 3 pear halves and add them to the blender with a few of the reserved whole basil leaves. Puree until very smooth. Strain through a coarse-mesh sieve into a small saucepan. Add salt and pepper to taste and heat. Halve the remaining pears lengthwise. Slice the turkey and serve it with the pear quarters, pear sauce, and basil sprigs for garnish.

Serves 6

CTC	Total Carbs	Fiber	Total Fat	Sat Fat	Protein	Calories
13.29	15.88	2.59	2.60	.60	40.83	255

brined turkey roast with sausage and leeks

Meats that tend to dry out during cooking increasingly are candidates for brining these days, with pork and poultry at the head of the line. I've used turkey sausages here so the dish can be prepared in kosher kitchens and because they contain less saturated fat than pork sausage. This is a kind of 3-in-1 offering: juicy slices of turkey, plump sausages, and caramelized leeks. Italian-style turkey sausages can be found in the fresh poultry section of most supermarkets. Many brands are preservative- and nitrite-free.

1	all-natural fresh turkey breast (6 pounds)
6	leeks
8	hot Italian-style turkey sausages (about 1 pound)

Up to 1 day before you plan to serve, place the turkey and enough cold water to cover in a large pot. Add 1 cup kosher salt and stir to dissolve. Cover and refrigerate for 8 to 12 hours.

Preheat the oven to 350°F.

Remove the turkey from the brine and pat it dry with paper towels. Season the turkey with freshly ground black pepper. Remove the pop-up timer, if there is one.

Remove the roots from the leeks and halve them lengthwise. Wash well between the layers to remove any dirt. Pat the leeks dry with paper towels and place them side by side, cut sides down, in a large, shallow roasting pan. Place the turkey on the leeks and tightly cover with foil.

Roast the turkey for about 1 hour and 30 minutes. Remove the foil and place the sausages around the turkey. Roast for 40 minutes longer, or until the temperature on an instant-read thermometer inserted in the thickest part reaches 150°F. Remove the roasting pan from the oven and transfer the leeks, sausages, and turkey to a warm platter. Cover with foil to keep warm.

Pour 1 cup boiling water into the roasting pan and scrape up any browned bits. Pour the pan juices through a sieve into a small saucepan. Bring to a boil and cook for several minutes until syrupy, adding salt and pepper to taste. Present the turkey to your guests, then slice it. Serve the turkey with the sausages, leeks, and hot pan juices.

Serves 8

nutritionist's note: Using turkey sausage instead of pork sausage saves 100 calories and 5 grams of saturated fat.

CTC	Total Carbs	Fiber	Total Fat	Sat Fat	Protein	Calories
9.06	10.26	1.20	9.49	2.30	63.09	387

holiday turkey with clove-studded oranges

This succulent bird gets its moist texture from quick brining and slow roasting. Its delicate fragrance and flavor come from stuffing the cavity with festive pomanders, once used for medicinal and household purposes. Instead, I've put these clove-studded oranges to good culinary use.

1	fresh turkey (14 pounds)
4	large oranges
2	tablespoons whole cloves

Remove the giblets and reserve for making stock. Discard the liver. Place the turkey in a pot large enough to accommodate it. Add cold water to cover. Add 1 cup kosher salt and stir to dissolve. Cover the turkey and brine it for 2 hours at room temperature, turning several times.

Meanwhile, wash 2 oranges and stud them each with 40 cloves.

Preheat the oven to 350°F.

Remove the turkey from the brine and pat it dry with paper towels. Place the pomanders in the cavity, then truss the turkey with string to secure the wings and hold the legs together. Season the turkey with freshly ground black pepper. Tightly cover the breast with foil. Roast the turkey for 2 hours.

Meanwhile, place the giblets in a saucepan, add 4 cups water, ½ tablespoon cloves, and bring to a boil. Skim any foam, reduce the heat to medium, and simmer for 30 minutes. Strain through a fine-mesh sieve. Return the liquid to the saucepan and simmer until it is reduced to 2 cups. Set aside.

After 2 hours, remove the foil from the turkey and raise the oven temperature to 400°F. Cook about 30 minutes longer, basting frequently with pan drippings, until the temperature on an instant-read thermometer inserted in the thigh reaches 165°F. Transfer to a board and let it rest for 15 minutes.

Pour off the fat from the pan. Pour in the reduced stock, scrape up any browned bits, and strain the pan juices through a sieve into a clean saucepan. Grate the zest of the remaining 2 oranges and add it to the stock. Squeeze the juice of these oranges and add to the stock. Bring to a boil, then reduce the heat and simmer until syrupy and reduced to about 1½ cups. Add salt and pepper to taste.

Remove the pomanders from the turkey and cut them each into 6 wedges. Carve the turkey as desired. Serve the turkey with the pomanders for decoration and the hot gravy.

Serves 10

CTC	Total Carbs	Fiber	Total Fat	Sat Fat	Protein	Calories
3.20	3.54	.34	7.49	2.32	61.67	344

fish and shellfish

Dennis Sweeney, one of my business associates, is fond of saying that, "eating fish is a matter of scale!" At no time has this been more true. No sooner has one branch of the government urged us to consume more fish, then another has cautioned us not to eat too much because of harmful PCBs, mercury, pesticides, and environmental pollutants. Meanwhile, chefs are refusing to serve certain species because they're being fished to extinction.

On top of all that, we're now being warned that farmed fish, much like cattle in feedlots, are loaded with antibiotics and other chemicals and living in unclean environments. There are additional cautions for pregnant women and small children about mercury in tuna, shark, swordfish, and king mackerel.

But fish *is* good for you. Inherently low in calories and fat, fish contains many beneficial nutrients, including vitamins A and D and omega-3 fatty acids, which can help lower blood levels of the harmful lipoproteins (aka LDL cholesterol) that contribute to heart disease. Omega-3 fatty acids can also help boost the immune system. We believe low-carbers should feel free to fill up on fish—just choose wild fish instead of farmed, whenever possible. Wild salmon and arctic char in particular contain fewer calories and are lower in saturated fat than farm-raised. However, women who are pregnant or wish to become pregnant should consult their doctors about mercury levels in fish and what intake may be appropriate.

All fish provide a great source of protein. White-fleshed fish such as halibut, cod, and sole are carb free, extremely low in saturated fat, and have a mere 25 calories per ounce. So-called fatty fish such as salmon and bluefish are full of heart-healthy omega-3 fatty acids. Tuna and swordfish, the meatier fish, have an imperceptible amount of fat and saturated fat, and about 35 calories per ounce. Shellfish contains about 1 gram of carbohydrates per ounce and little saturated fat.

The current thinking about safety seems to be that you're better off eating fish than fatty meat and that you're better off eating lots of different kinds of fish, just as we're advised to eats lots of different kinds of vegetables. In that spirit, you will enjoy the recipes included in this chapter, featuring a wide variety of fish and shellfish.

Choose your fish supplier with care. A market that sells a great deal of fish, with high turnover, usually has fresher products and a wider range of choice. A market that will fillet whole fish to order usually has better quality than those that don't. Prepackaged fish in supermarkets worries me because I can't look into the fish's eyes to see if they're clear and shiny, as they should be, and I can't always see the skin or the surface of the fish to see if it's glistening, firm, and compact. It's also hard to smell fish through a tightly wrapped package to determine its freshness. Great fresh fish smells like the sea.

Many of the preparations in this chapter are interchangeable. For example, the crust on the Pesto-Pistachio Chilean Sea Bass (page 166) is also fabulous on salmon; swordfish can be substituted successfully for the bass in the Striped Bass with Bacon and Cabbage (page 174).

There's no need for fancy (and often fat- and carb-laden) sauces either. These recipes maximize the unique flavor and the singular texture of each variety of fish rather than overwhelm its virtues.

Haven't cooked much fish at home in the past? May these recipes inspire you to do it often in the future.

sautéed shrimp with bell pepper confetti

With its tiny cubes of colorful bell peppers, this dish looks like a party. The peppers are slowly steamed in a bath of olive oil and water. This flavors the oil and softens the peppers luxuriously. The mixture makes a great topping for grilled swordfish or halibut as well.

3	medium bell peppers, 1 red, 1 yellow, and 1 green
6	tablespoons garlic-flavored olive oil
36	large shrimp in their shells (about 1¾ pounds)

Halve the peppers lengthwise and remove the seeds. Cut the peppers into ¼"-wide strips, then into ¼" cubes, making them as uniform as possible. Place them in a medium saucepan with a cover. Add 4 tablespoons of the oil, ½ cup water, a large pinch of salt, and ¼ teaspoon whole black peppercorns. Bring just to a boil, immediately reduce the heat, and cover the pan. Simmer until the peppers are soft but still retain their shape, about 20 minutes. Remove from the heat.

Meanwhile, peel the shrimp and discard the shells. In a large nonstick skillet over medium heat, heat the remaining 2 tablespoons oil. Add the shrimp and cook, stirring frequently, until the shrimp are opaque and just firm to the touch, about 3 minutes. Add salt and freshly ground black pepper to taste.

When ready to serve, heat the peppers until hot, adding salt to taste. Divide the shrimp among four large flat soup plates or dinner plates and spoon the warm peppers and liquid over the shrimp. Serve immediately.

Serves 4

CTC	Total Carbs	Fiber	Total Fat	Sat Fat	Protein	Calories
4.57	5.83	1.26	23.30	3.31	34.98	377

basil shrimp and crispy pancetta

Shrimp shells are boiled and used as a simple stock that helps meld the diverse flavors. This also makes a great first course and is delicious made with fresh sage as well.

4 ounces pancetta, cut into ¼" dice
24 jumbo shrimp in their shells (about 2 pounds)
16 large fresh basil leaves

Put the pancetta and 1 cup water in a small saucepan and bring to a boil. Boil 1 minute and drain off the water. Transfer the pancetta to a very large nonstick skillet. Cook over medium heat until the fat is rendered and the pancetta starts turning golden and crisp, about 5 minutes. Remove from the heat and set aside.

Meanwhile, peel and devein the shrimp, leaving the tails on. Put the shells in a large saucepan and add cold water to cover, about 8 cups. Boil for 10 minutes. Pour off the shrimp broth and reserve. Discard the shells.

Add the shrimp to the pancetta and cook over medium-high heat, stirring once or twice, until they begin to turn opaque, about 2 minutes. Meanwhile, coarsely tear 12 basil leaves and add them to the pan. Toss gently, cover, reduce the heat to low, and cook until the shrimp are fully cooked, 1 to 2 minutes. Add coarsely ground black pepper and ¼ cup or more of the shrimp broth. Cook, uncovered and stirring with a wooden spoon, for 1 minute longer. Garnish with the remaining basil leaves and serve immediately.

Serves 4

CTC	Total Carbs	Fiber	Total Fat	Sat Fat	Protein	Calories
1.69	1.77	.08	15.35	4.66	45.58	338

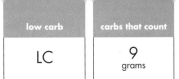
shrimp in coconut-tomato sauce

When it works, "fusion cuisine" means taking ingredients from disparate parts of the world and combining them in new and exciting ways. Here's a surprising dish with elements from Italy and Southeast Asia that tastes like it came from neither place, but whose flavors coalesce wondrously.

32   large shrimp in their shells (about 1½ pounds)
1⅓ cups light coconut milk
1⅓ cups good-quality marinara sauce

Remove the shrimp from their shells, discard the shells, and set aside the shrimp.

In a very large nonstick skillet over medium heat, combine the coconut milk and marinara sauce. Cook, stirring constantly, just until well blended. Add salt and freshly ground black pepper to taste. Bring the mixture to a boil and add the shrimp. Cook over high heat, stirring constantly, until the shrimp turn pink, 5 to 6 minutes. (Be careful not to overcook.) Using a slotted spoon, immediately transfer the shrimp to 4 warm shallow soup bowls.

Over high heat, cook the sauce, stirring constantly, until thickened, about 2 minutes longer. Pour the sauce over the shrimp and serve immediately.

Serves 4

nutritionist's note: Using light coconut milk instead of the more expected heavy cream saves you 14 grams of saturated fat.

CTC	Total Carbs	Fiber	Total Fat	Sat Fat	Protein	Calories
8.82	10.15	1.33	8.65	4.70	30.96	248

steamed mussels, singapore-style

Mussels take kindly to all sorts of flavors, but this marriage is unique. Slightly Asian, it produces a light, yet intriguingly creamy bowl of steaming shellfish and is completely different from the flavor profile in the preceding recipe, although it also uses coconut milk as one of its 3 ingredients. You should be able to find these large, plump mussels in most fish stores.

3   pounds large green-lipped New Zealand mussels
1¾   cups light coconut milk
2   bunches fresh cilantro

Scrub the mussels, removing any beards, if necessary. Discard any mussels that are open.

In a food processor, combine the coconut milk and 1½ cups water. Cut the leaves from the cilantro stems and finely chop enough leaves to get 1 packed cup. Add the chopped cilantro to the food processor, along with a pinch of salt and ground white pepper. Process until the cilantro is in tiny pieces.

Place the coconut-cilantro mixture in a 4-quart pot with a cover. Bring the mixture to a boil and add the mussels. Quickly cover the pot and cook the mussels, shaking the pot back and forth frequently to distribute the mussels, for 6 to 8 minutes. When the mussels have opened (discard any that haven't), remove them with a slotted spoon and transfer them to 4 large warm bowls.

Continue to boil the liquid in the pot until the sauce thickens, about 2 minutes longer. Pour the sauce over the mussels and serve immediately.

Serves 4

CTC	Total Carbs	Fiber	Total Fat	Sat Fat	Protein	Calories
9.46	9.95	.49	9.90	6.00	22.33	220

chilean sea bass with melted leeks

Chilean sea bass is thick, flaky, snow-white, mild, and juicy. It is especially lovable under a buttery sauce of "melted" leeks—which provides a gentle and sophisticated accompaniment. If you're concerned about overfishing of this species, substitute very thick pieces of cod.

4	large leeks (about 1¼ pounds)
2	tablespoons + 2½ teaspoons unsalted butter
4	thick Chilean sea bass fillets (7 ounces each)

Remove the dark green parts from the leeks and discard them. Slice the white parts of the leeks paper-thin. Wash the leeks well, making sure to remove any dirt. Pat the leeks dry with paper towels.

In a large saucepan over medium-high heat, melt 2 tablespoons of the butter. Add the leeks, 6 tablespoons water, ¼ teaspoon salt, and ground white pepper. Bring to a quick boil, then reduce the heat to a simmer, cover, and cook for 25 minutes.

Add ¼ cup water to the saucepan, cover again, and cook 10 minutes longer. (The leeks should be very soft and form a *fondue*, which means "melted.") Remove the saucepan from the heat and set it aside.

Season the fish with salt and ground white pepper. In a very large nonstick skillet over medium-high heat, melt the remaining 2½ teaspoons butter. Add the fish to the skillet and cook until golden, making sure the fish is opaque throughout, about 3 minutes per side. (Be careful not to overcook.)

Gently reheat the leek fondue and pour it over the hot fish in the pan. Sprinkle with coarse salt and serve.

Serves 4

CTC	Total Carbs	Fiber	Total Fat	Sat Fat	Protein	Calories
14.01	16.05	2.04	12.30	6.09	36.77	325

pesto-pistachio chilean sea bass

This is a showstopper: brilliantly white fish blanketed with a crunchy, green crust. Buy a really good pesto sauce from your market's refrigerated section. You can substitute a thick fillet of halibut, which is another firm, white fish, or even a thick fillet of salmon.

2½ pounds Chilean sea bass, in 1 piece
1 cup shelled unsalted pistachios
¾ cup prepared pesto

Preheat the oven to 400°F.

Line a rimmed baking sheet with parchment paper or foil.

Using tweezers, remove any bones running down the center of the fish. Lightly season both sides of the fish with salt and place it on the baking sheet.

In a food processor, process the pistachios until coarsely ground. (Do not overprocess; you want small, discernible pieces, not powder.)

Thickly spread the pesto on top of the fish to coat it completely, draining most of the oil from the pesto as you go. Dust the fish with freshly ground black pepper. Pack the pistachios onto the pesto to cover evenly and press down lightly to obtain a thick nut crust.

Bake the fish for 35 to 40 minutes, or until the fish reaches the desired doneness. (Do not overcook; it is important to keep the fish moist and juicy.) Remove the fish from the oven, transfer it to a large warm platter, and serve immediately.

Serves 6

nutritionist's note: While shopping for prepared pesto, compare labels and use the brand with the least amount of fat. FYI, pistachios in their shell make a great snack. Thirty of them have only 5 grams of CTC and shelling them yourself makes them last a long time.

CTC	Total Carbs	Fiber	Total Fat	Sat Fat	Protein	Calories
4.47	7.77	3.30	18.85	3.47	43.65	377

lettuce-wrapped cod with herb oil

Years before the low-carb movement, this dish was fashionable among obsessive calorie-counters who frequented fancy French restaurants. It looks and taste great, and the edible green wrapper of lettuce not only seals in the juices, but it also adds to its healthful presentation.

4   cod fillets (8 ounces each), without skin
8   large green leaf lettuce leaves
6   tablespoons basil- or rosemary-flavored olive oil

Using tweezers, remove any bones from the fish. Lightly season the fish with salt and freshly ground black pepper and set aside.

Bring a large pot of salted water to a boil. Add the lettuce leaves and boil until just pliable, about 1 minute. Remove the leaves immediately and place them in a colander under cold running water, being careful not to tear the leaves. Pat the leaves dry with paper towels.

Brush 1 teaspoon of the oil on each piece of fish. Wrap each fillet in 2 lettuce leaves, pressing down tightly and completely enclosing the fish.

Fill a large pot with a fitted lid and a flat steamer basket halfway with water and bring to a boil. Place the wrapped fish in the steamer basket in a single layer, cover, and cook over medium heat for 15 to 20 minutes.

While the fish is cooking, gently heat the remaining oil in a small saucepan with 3 tablespoons water and a liberal pinch of salt. Keep warm. Carefully remove the fish from the steamer and transfer it to plates. Drizzle the warm sauce over the fish and serve immediately.

Serves 4

CTC	Total Carbs	Fiber	Total Fat	Sat Fat	Protein	Calories
.21	.63	.42	21.83	3.04	40.67	368

baked cod in crispy grape leaves

Lemon-kissed olive oil and briny grape leaves impart a distinctly Mediterranean air to this dish. Grapes leaves are sold packed in brine, and you can find them in Middle Eastern food stores or near the olives in your supermarket. Keep the leaves on the fish when you serve it because they are crisp and delicious.

6   thick cod fillets (7 ounces each), without skin
6   tablespoons lemon-flavored olive oil
10 large grape leaves in brine

Preheat the oven to 450°F.

Using tweezers, remove any bones from the fish. Coat each fillet with 2 teaspoons of the oil and season with freshly ground black pepper.

Remove the grape leaves from the brine and rinse them thoroughly under cold water. Pat them very dry with paper towels. Remove any stems or tough veins. On a clean surface, place 2 grape leaves, with the ends overlapping slightly and the tips of the leaves pointed in opposite directions to make an elongated grape leaf. Place 1 fish fillet in the center and wrap tightly, tucking in the ends of the leaves to make a tight, neat package. Repeat with the remaining fillets. Roll the remaining 2 grape leaves into a tight roll and cut across into very fine strips.

In a very large skillet over medium-high heat, heat 1½ tablespoons oil. Sear the fish bundles for 20 to 30 seconds on each side so they get crispy. Spread ½ tablespoon oil in the center of a rimmed baking sheet and place the fish bundles on the sheet. Scatter the strips of grape leaves around the fish.

Bake for 8 to 10 minutes, depending on the thickness of the fish. Remove the fish from the oven and transfer it to warm plates. Scatter with the now crispy strips of grape leaves and drizzle additional lemon oil around the fish. Serve immediately.

Serves 4

CTC	Total Carbs	Fiber	Total Fat	Sat Fat	Protein	Calories
1.17	1.17	0	22.53	1.04	35.75	350

grouper en papillote with oranges and tapenade

This highly theatrical dish is a cinch to make. Baked in puffed-up packets of foil or parchment, this can be presented to your guests, then plated back in the kitchen. The ingredients make their own salty and slightly sweet sauce right in the parchment packages. Tapenade is a black olive paste that can be purchased in jars. This is also great made with halibut and blood oranges, when in season.

4	grouper fillets (7 ounces each), without skin
½	cup black olive tapenade
4	large oranges

Preheat the oven to 375°F.

Cut four 30" lengths of parchment paper or foil. Fold each in half lengthwise. Place a fish fillet on each, slightly off center. Spread the entire surface of the fish fillets with a thin layer of the tapenade. Grate the zest of enough oranges to get 2 teaspoons. Sprinkle each fish with ½ teaspoon zest.

With a small, very sharp knife, pare away the skin and all of the white pith from the oranges and cut them into thin slices, being sure to remove the seeds. Place overlapping slices of oranges on top of each piece of fish, along with any accumulated orange juice.

Fold the parchment over the fish, crimping the edges tightly to make airtight packages and rolling up the edges as you go. (The shape should look like a half-moon.) Place the packets on a baking sheet and bake them for 20 minutes. Remove the packets from the oven, cut them open, remove the fish and all of the juices, and serve immediately.

Serves 4

nutritionist's note: The polyphenols contained in olives are antioxidant compounds that can help keep your arteries clear. Buy an olive tapenade that is preservative free.

CTC	Total Carbs	Fiber	Total Fat	Sat Fat	Protein	Calories
15.45	18.59	3.14	11.10	.66	42.50	344

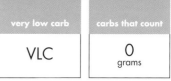
prosciutto-wrapped halibut

The salty-gamey contrast of prosciutto provides just the right amount of interest to the sweet gentle flavor of halibut. I suggest that you use Italian rather than domestic prosciutto because it is generally moister and holds up better in the oven. You may substitute any firm white fish fillet, such as haddock or cod, that is about ½" thick.

6   halibut fillets (7 ounces each), without skin
8   tablespoons garlic-flavored olive oil
12   thin slices prosciutto (about 6 ounces)

Preheat the oven to 425°F.

Season the fish with freshly ground black pepper. With your fingers, apply a small amount of the oil to the halibut fillets. (You need just enough so the prosciutto will adhere.) Tightly wrap 2 slices of prosciutto around each fillet to cover and form a thick sausage shape.

In a large nonstick skillet over medium-high heat, heat a little of the oil. Add the fish and sear on all sides, 30 to 45 seconds per side.

Transfer the fish to a rimmed baking sheet and drizzle with the remaining oil. Bake for 10 to 12 minutes, or until the fish is just firm. Place the fish under the broiler, about 8" from the heat, and broil for 2 minutes to crisp the prosciutto a bit, if desired.

Transfer the fish to warm plates. If the fillets are thick, cut into thick slices on the bias and place in an overlapping fashion on each plate. Drizzle the fish with any pan juices, sprinkle with coarsely ground black pepper, and serve immediately.

Serves 6

CTC	Total Carbs	Fiber	Total Fat	Sat Fat	Protein	Calories
0	0	0	23.0	3.69	43.32	383

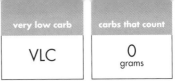
bay-steamed halibut with lemon oil

Trendy chefs are using the cooking technique of this recipe—gently cooking fish (or meat) with its seasoning in a tightly sealed wrapper. The flavors fuse together in a unique way and the fish cooks in its own juices. Be careful not to marinate the fish too long or it will taste "perfume-y." Bay leaves impart great flavor, but avoid eating them because the leaf or its stem could get stuck in your throat.

4	halibut steaks (8 ounces each)
16	whole bay leaves
8	teaspoons lemon-flavored olive oil

Place each piece of fish on a large square of plastic wrap and season with salt and freshly ground black pepper. Place 4 bay leaves side by side to cover one side of each steak and drizzle with 1 teaspoon of the oil. Tightly wrap the fish in plastic wrap and place it in the refrigerator for 3 to 4 hours, but no longer.

Fill a large pot with a tightly fitting lid and a steamer basket halfway with water and bring it to a boil. Place the wrapped fish in the steamer basket in the pot and cover tightly. Steam the fish until cooked through, 10 to 12 minutes, depending on the thickness of the fish.

Meanwhile, in a small bowl, mix together the remaining oil with a pinch of coarse salt.

Carefully remove the fish from the steamer and unwrap the packets. Discard the bay leaves and serve the fish immediately, drizzled with juices from packet and the remaining oil.

Serves 4

CTC	Total Carbs	Fiber	Total Fat	Sat Fat	Protein	Calories
0	.10	.10	14.53	1.95	47.17	330

sautéed snapper in champagne sauce

The pink-tinged sauce of this dish is both suave and simple. Just be sure to use a brut rose champagne because you want to avoid sweetness here.

6   red snapper fillets (8 ounces each), with skin
4   tablespoons + 1 teaspoon unsalted butter
1   cup brut rose champagne

Using tweezers, remove any bones from the fish. Lightly season the fish with salt and freshly ground white pepper. Make several crosshatch slits in the skin of each fillet to prevent the fish from curling up while cooking.

In each of 2 large nonstick skillets (big enough to hold the fish in one layer) over medium heat, melt 1½ tablespoons of the butter. Place 3 fillets, skin side up, in each skillet. Cook until the fish is opaque and lightly golden, about 2 minutes. Turn the fish over with a spatula, increase the heat a bit, and cook until the skin begins to crisp, about 3 minutes longer. Transfer the fish to a platter and loosely cover with foil.

Quickly combine the pan juices into 1 pan and add the champagne. Turn the heat to high and cook, stirring, until the liquid is reduced to ⅓ cup. Reduce the heat to a simmer and whisk the remaining butter into the sauce until thick and creamy. Add salt and pepper to taste, pour the sauce over the fish, and serve.

Serves 6

nutritionist's note: You can sip some leftover champagne with only 1.5 grams of CTC for every 4 ounces. Don't forget to chill it.

CTC	Total Carbs	Fiber	Total Fat	Sat Fat	Protein	Calories
.56	.56	0	10.98	5.74	40.85	300

lemon sole in burnt orange oil

You'll be amazed how much flavor can be coaxed from an orange, especially when you extract volatile oils from the skin, reduce the juices into a delectable sauce, and garnish the whole deal with orange segments.

5	medium juice oranges
¼	cup garlic- or herb-flavored olive oil
4	thick lemon sole fillets (7 ounces each), without skin

With a vegetable peeler, remove 8 long strips of the orange zest and reserve. Cut the rind and all pith off 4 of the oranges. Cut in between the membranes to release the orange segments. Set aside. Squeeze the juice of the remaining orange and set aside.

In a very large nonstick skillet over medium-high heat, heat the oil. Add the strips of orange zest. Just as the strips become dark brown, about 1 minute, remove them from the skillet with a slotted spoon and set them aside.

Sprinkle both sides of the fish with salt and pepper. Add the fish to the hot oil in the skillet and cook over medium heat on both sides until the fish is crisp and lightly browned, about 2 to 3 minutes per side. (You may need to cook the fish in 2 batches.) Remove the cooked fish to a warm platter and cover loosely with foil.

Add the orange segments and the orange juice to the oil in the skillet. Cook over high heat for 1 minute, add salt and freshly ground black pepper to taste, and pour the sauce over the fish. Garnish the fish with the burnt orange peel and serve immediately.

Serves 4

CTC	Total Carbs	Fiber	Total Fat	Sat Fat	Protein	Calories
14.55	17.74	3.19	16.88	2.41	42.10	390

striped bass with bacon and cabbage

This is my idea of cold-weather comfort food, but you can make it whenever the spirit moves you. I'd serve it with a light Pinot Noir or a robust Riesling from Alsace, both of which will enhance the smoky bacon overtones of this dish. Choose a nitrite-free bacon.

1   head savoy cabbage (about 1½ pounds)
3   ounces slab bacon
4   striped bass fillets (7 ounces each), without skin

Trim away any limp or damaged leaves from the cabbage and wash it well. Cut the cabbage in half through the stem end, then cut out the core. Place the cabbage, cut sides down, on a cutting board and use a large, sharp knife to slice across the width into ¼" slices.

Cut the bacon into evenly sized ¼" cubes. Transfer the cubes to a 12" nonstick skillet with a cover. Cook over medium heat, stirring often, until the fat is rendered and the bacon begins to crisp, about 3 minutes.

Add the cabbage, ½ cup water, ½ teaspoon coarse salt, and freshly ground black pepper to the skillet. Cook over medium-high heat, stirring frequently, for about 10 minutes. Add another ½ cup water, reduce the heat to medium, cover the skillet, and cook until the cabbage is browned and soft, about 30 minutes. If the cabbage begins to stick, add a little more water.

Season the fish with salt and freshly ground black pepper. Place the fish on the cabbage in the skillet. Add ¼ cup water and cover the skillet. Cook until the fish is cooked through, 10 to 12 minutes.

Using a spatula, divide the cabbage and fish among 4 warm large plates. Drizzle with any hot pan juices and serve immediately.

Serves 4

nutritionist's note: Here's a great example of how a little bacon can add a lot of flavor while still keeping within our saturated fat goals.

CTC	Total Carbs	Fiber	Total Fat	Sat Fat	Protein	Calories
8.50	17.29	8.79	14.02	4.08	46.91	375

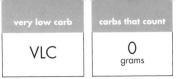

sautéed striped bass with basil sauce

My secret technique is to freeze the olive oil required in this dish so that the sauce takes on a light, emulsified quality. Just be sure to allow plenty of extra time for this step. You must use impeccably fresh basil, first-class olive oil, and pristine fish—there's no place for inferior ingredients to hide.

5   tablespoons extra-virgin or garlic-flavored olive oil
2   large bunches basil
4   striped bass fillets (7 ounces each), without skin

Place 3 tablespoons of the oil in a custard cup or ramekin and freeze until hard.

Coarsely chop enough basil to get 3 packed cups. Reserve some small sprigs for garnish. Bring a pot of salted water to a boil. Add the basil and boil for 2½ minutes. Drain the basil immediately and transfer it to a blender with the frozen oil and 3 to 4 tablespoons water. Process until thick and creamy. It should make about ¾ cup. Transfer the mixture to a small saucepan and add salt and freshly ground black pepper to taste.

Season the fish with salt and pepper. In a large nonstick skillet over medium-high heat, heat the remaining 2 tablespoons oil until hot. Add the fish and cook, turning once, until it becomes opaque and golden on both sides, about 2 to 3 minutes per side. Serve immediately with the gently reheated sauce and garnish with the remaining basil sprigs.

Serves 4

CTC	Total Carbs	Fiber	Total Fat	Sat Fat	Protein	Calories
.14	1.38	1.24	22.31	1.02	35.98	351

swordfish *peperonata*

Peperonata is a yielding compote of colorful peppers that stew in extra-virgin olive oil and their own sweet juices. Terrific served warm atop juicy swordfish, it is also delicious at room temperature or chilled.

4	swordfish steaks (7 ounces each)
¼	cup extra-virgin olive oil
4	medium bell peppers, 2 red or orange and 2 yellow

Coat each fish steak with ½ tablespoon of the oil and freshly ground black pepper. Set aside while you prepare the *peperonata*.

Cut the peppers into long, thin strips, no more than ¼" wide, making sure to remove all of the seeds.

In a large nonstick skillet over medium-high heat, heat the remaining 2 tablespoons oil. Add the pepper strips, ½ teaspoon whole black peppercorns, and ½ teaspoon coarse salt. Reduce the heat to low and cook, stirring occasionally, until the peppers are soft and lightly browned, about 20 minutes. Remove the peppers from the heat and set aside.

Heat an iron-ribbed grill pan or nonstick skillet over medium-high heat until hot. Add the fish and cook on both sides, about 3 minutes per side, until the fish is browned on the outside and moist inside. Meanwhile, briefly warm the peppers. Serve the fish with the warm *peperonata* on top.

Serves 4

nutritionist's note: The olive oil in this dish gives the peppers a nutritional boost. Fat allows your body to better absorb the beta-carotene found in bell peppers.

CTC	Total Carbs	Fiber	Total Fat	Sat Fat	Protein	Calories
5.39	7.65	2.26	22.18	4.03	40.33	392

sautéed turbot with asparagus and asparagus velouté

You use fresh asparagus two ways here, as a vegetable and as a velvety sauce that you whip up quickly in a blender. Cod or tilapia is a good substitute for the turbot.

1½ pounds medium asparagus
2 tablespoons + 2 teaspoons unsalted butter
4 turbot fillets (8 ounces each), as thick as possible

Trim the top 3" of the asparagus and set these tips aside. Trim 1" from the bottom of the stalks and discard. Peel the stalks with a vegetable peeler and cut into 1" pieces. Transfer the asparagus pieces to a saucepan with enough salted water to cover. Bring the water to a boil, reduce the heat, and simmer until the asparagus is very soft, about 10 minutes. Using a slotted spoon, transfer the asparagus to a blender. Add ¾ to 1 cup cooking liquid to the blender and process until smooth. Add 2 tablespoons of the butter and continue to process until very smooth. Add salt and freshly ground black pepper to taste and blend.

Bring a small pot of salted water to a boil. Add the asparagus tips and cook until just tender, about 5 minutes. Drain, set aside, and keep warm.

Meanwhile, season the fish with salt and pepper. In a very large nonstick skillet over medium-high heat, melt the remaining 2 teaspoons butter. Add the fish to the skillet and cook until golden, about 3 minutes. Carefully turn the fish over and cook it until golden on the other side, about 2 minutes longer. Turn the fish again, cover the pan, and cook until the fish reaches the desired doneness, just beginning to flake, about 3 minutes longer, depending on the thickness.

Spoon some of the gently reheated sauce on each plate. Top with the fish and asparagus tips. Spoon a little of the sauce on top and serve immediately.

Serves 4

nutritionist's note: Feel free to double the asparagus—4 stalks have only 1.5 grams of CTC, no saturated fat, and only 15 calories.

CTC	Total Carbs	Fiber	Total Fat	Sat Fat	Protein	Calories
4.13	7.73	3.60	10.71	5.52	46.70	313

arctic char with dill and vermouth

Artic char is the northernmost fish we eat. It bears resemblance to salmon, and the two often can be interchanged in recipes. Like salmon, it now is farmed, and farmed char has more calories and fat than wild arctic char. For this recipe, I prefer wild arctic char, if you can find it. I've provided the nutritional analysis for both farmed and wild so you can see the differences for yourself.

4	wild arctic char fillets (7 ounces each), with skin
1	cup dry vermouth
1	bunch fresh dill

Run your fingers over the fillets to locate any bones and remove them using tweezers. Place the fillets in one layer in a shallow baking dish. Pour the vermouth over the fish.

Finely chop about ¾ cup dill and scatter it over the fish. Sprinkle ground white pepper and some fine sea salt over the fish. Cover and refrigerate for 1 hour.

Preheat the oven to 425°F.

Remove the fish from the marinade. Place the fish, skin side down, on a rimmed baking sheet. Bake for 12 to 13 minutes, depending on the thickness of the fish. Remove the fish from the oven and serve immediately, garnished with tufts of the remaining dill.

Serves 4

wild arctic char

CTC	Total Carbs	Fiber	Total Fat	Sat Fat	Protein	Calories
.28	.32	.04	5.38	.84	40.74	227

farmed

CTC	Total Carbs	Fiber	Total Fat	Sat Fat	Protein	Calories
.28	.32	.04	24.23	4.29	36.97	380

wasabi salmon

It takes just 3 minutes to prepare this dish, but its memory will linger. The wasabi coating is creamy, pungent, and very modern. The salmon can be cut into 4 fillets before baking, or you can use a large 2-pound piece cut from the center of the fish and portion it after baking for a more dramatic presentation. Be sure to use wild salmon; although it is a bit pricier, it has fewer health risks than farmed salmon.

4 wild salmon fillets (8 ounces each), with skin
3 tablespoons wasabi powder
¾ cup light mayonnaise

Preheat the oven to 450°F.

Line a rimmed baking sheet with parchment paper or foil.

Using tweezers, remove any bones from the fish. Season the fish with salt and freshly ground black pepper.

In a bowl, mix the wasabi powder with 2 to 2½ tablespoons water to form a smooth, thick paste. Add the mayonnaise and mix thoroughly. Add a pinch of salt and pepper. Spread the mixture on top of the fish to cover completely.

Place the fish on the baking sheet and bake until the fish is lightly golden but still moist, about 15 minutes, depending on the thickness of the fish. (Do not overcook.) Using a spatula, remove the fish from its skin and discard the skin. Serve immediately.

Serves 4

nutritionist's note: Farmed salmon is carb free, yet it has an additional gram of saturated fat and 10 more calories per ounce than wild salmon.

CTC	Total Carbs	Fiber	Total Fat	Sat Fat	Protein	Calories
4.13	4.13	0	26.90	4.67	34.85	396

salmon steaks with cornichon vinaigrette

If you've read about "warm vinaigrette" dressings and wondered how to make them, here's the answer. In no time at all, you get crispy salmon in a heady, sweet-and-briny sauce and next-to-zero carbs. Cornichons, tiny French pickled cucumbers, are available in most supermarkets and fancy food stores.

5	tablespoons extra-virgin olive oil
½	cup French cornichons, with their pickling liquid
4	wild salmon steaks (8 ounces each), with skin

To prepare the vinaigrette, in a small saucepan, combine 4 tablespoons of the oil and 4 tablespoons pickling juice from the cornichons. Finely mince enough cornichons so that you have 6 tablespoons. Add them to the saucepan with a grinding of black pepper. Warm the mixture gently over low heat for 30 seconds and set it aside.

Season both sides of the salmon with salt and pepper. In a large nonstick skillet over high heat, heat the remaining 1 tablespoon oil. Place the salmon steaks in the skillet and cook until they are browned and crisp on one side, about 3 minutes. Carefully turn the salmon over with a spatula and cook to the desired doneness, 2 to 3 minutes longer. (Do not overcook.)

Remove the skin from the salmon and place the salmon steaks on individual plates or a large platter. Pour the vinaigrette into the same skillet that you just used to cook the salmon, to warm it slightly. Pour over the fish and serve immediately.

Serves 4

CTC	Total Carbs	Fiber	Total Fat	Sat Fat	Protein	Calories
1.05	1.50	.45	28.28	3.95	33.73	396

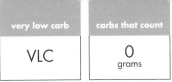
crispy salmon with pancetta and sage

When people ask me for an example of a 3-ingredient recipe, this is usually the one I give, where the whole is more than the sum of its parts. Pancetta is an Italian version of spiced-cured, but un-smoked bacon. In this recipe, the pancetta both lubricates and flavors the salmon. This dish, enhanced with fresh sage, is like a salmon club sandwich without the bread.

4	ounces pancetta, sliced ⅛" thick
4	wild salmon fillets (7 ounces each), with skin
24	fresh sage leaves

In a large nonstick skillet, arrange the pancetta in a single layer. Cook the pancetta over low heat until most of the fat is rendered and the pancetta is just beginning to crisp. (You may need to do this in 2 batches.) Remove the pancetta with a spatula and let it cool for 5 minutes. Leave the rendered fat in the skillet off the heat.

Using tweezers, remove any bones from the salmon. You may remove the skin if you wish, but I prefer to leave it on. Holding a small, sharp knife on the bias, cut 2 deep slits across the width of each piece of fish to make 2 pockets. Do not cut all the way across or all the way down.

Place a crisp pancetta slice and 3 whole sage leaves in each pocket, allowing the edges of the sage and pancetta to show. Reheat the fat in the skillet over medium heat. Season the fish with salt and freshly ground black pepper and place the fish, pocket side down, in the skillet. Cook until the fish begins to brown and get crisp, about 3 minutes. Turn the salmon and finish cooking to the desired doneness, about 2 to 3 minutes longer. The salmon should be crispy on top and moist inside. Serve immediately, skin side down. Be sure to leave the fat in the pan.

Serves 4

CTC	Total Carbs	Fiber	Total Fat	Sat Fat	Protein	Calories
.01	.13	.12	22.95	5.72	41.90	384

pink-and-white "osso buco"

Translated literally from Italian, osso buco means "bone with hole." It usually refers to the bone in the center of a braised veal shank. Here, a big sea scallop, centered in a rosy steak of salmon, simulates that bone. You can swap colors by centering a piece of salmon in a halibut steak and follow the same recipe procedures. I've provided the nutritional data for both versions.

4   wild salmon steaks (7 ounces each), without skin (or halibut steaks)

4   large sea scallops (or four 1-ounce pieces of wild salmon)

4   slices nitrite-free bacon

Preheat the oven to 400°F.

Using tweezers, remove any bones from the salmon steaks, including the small center bone. Insert 1 sea scallop between the flaps of each salmon steak, filling in the area where the little center bone was. Cut off a 1" piece from the end of one flap so that you can easily wrap the flaps around the sea scallop. The goal is to make a tight, round shape.

Wrap 1 bacon slice around the edges of each fish package (as though you were replacing the skin) and secure it tightly with several toothpicks. Place the salmon on a rimmed baking sheet. Sprinkle with salt. Bake for 10 minutes, or until the fish is cooked to the desired doneness. (Do not overcook.) Sprinkle with coarsely cracked black pepper.

Serves 4

wild salmon with scallops

CTC	Total Carbs	Fiber	Total Fat	Sat Fat	Protein	Calories
.35	.35	0	18.69	3.96	45.87	365

halibut with wild salmon

CTC	Total Carbs	Fiber	Total Fat	Sat Fat	Protein	Calories
0	0	0	12.18	2.9	49.42	321

tuna steak "au poivre"

This is a lighter riff on steak au poivre. It has the punch of black pepper offset by the sweet acidity of balsamic vinegar. The sauce reduces to something that looks like chocolatey ketchup and is also great over swordfish, pork, chicken, or even hamburgers!

½ cup good-quality balsamic vinegar
4 tuna medallions, 1" thick (8 ounces each)
3 tablespoons unsalted butter, chilled

In a small nonreactive saucepan, bring the vinegar to a boil. Reduce the heat and simmer until the vinegar is reduced to 3 tablespoons. Remove the saucepan from the heat and set it aside.

Crush 2 tablespoons black peppercorns and press firmly into one side of each tuna medallion. Lightly sprinkle the tuna with salt. In a 12" nonstick skillet over high heat, melt 1 tablespoon of the butter. Add the fish, pepper side down, and cook for 3 minutes. Turn the fish over and cook it until it is still very pink in the center, 45 seconds to 1 minute. Remove the fish to a serving plate and keep warm under tented foil.

Quickly add the remaining 2 tablespoons butter and the reduced vinegar to the skillet and cook over high heat, whisking constantly, until thick, about 1 minute. Pour the sauce around the fish and serve.

Serves 4

nutritionist's note: By switching from beef to tuna, this recipe saves you 15 grams of fat (6 of them saturated fat) and 135 calories per serving.

CTC	Total Carbs	Fiber	Total Fat	Sat Fat	Protein	Calories
4.01	4.01	0	10.79	5.91	53.11	341

grilled tuna with orange-mint salsa

Here's another way of peppering a tuna steak, this time with pungent white peppercorns, which you can find in specialty food stores, kitchenware shops, and many supermarkets. The cooling salsa of fresh orange and mint offers a terrific flavor punch. Make sure to keep the tuna sushi-style rare in order to really experience all the elements of the dish.

4	small juice oranges
1	bunch spearmint or peppermint
4	tuna steaks (8 ounces each)

Peel the oranges with a sharp knife. Cut the oranges into ¼" slices, then into ¼" cubes. Finely chop the mint to get ¼ cup. In a bowl, combine the mint and oranges with a pinch of salt and freshly ground black pepper and mix gently. Refrigerate for 30 minutes to 1 hour.

Press ½ teaspoon very coarsely ground white pepper into one side of each tuna steak. Lightly sprinkle the tuna with salt. Spray a large nonstick skillet with cooking spray and heat the skillet over medium-high heat until hot. Place the tuna, pepper side down, in the skillet and cook on both sides until the fish is seared on the outside but still quite rare in the center, about 1 minute per side. Serve the hot tuna with the cold orange-mint salsa.

Serves 4

CTC	Total Carbs	Fiber	Total Fat	Sat Fat	Protein	Calories
9.09	11.52	2.43	2.28	.55	53.96	291

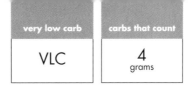
sautéed tuna provencal

This hearty recipe, adapted from something I tried on a trip to the south of France, tastes almost meat-like and is sure to become a favorite. Serve this with a glass of rose wine for a lovely lunch.

2   cans (4⅜ ounces each) skinless and boneless sardines in oil
1   cup good-quality marinara sauce
4   tuna steaks (7 ounces each)

Drain 2 teaspoons oil from each can of sardines and discard the rest of the oil. Set it aside.

In a saucepan, combine the sardines and marinara sauce. Add a large pinch of salt and lots of freshly ground black pepper. Bring the mixture just to a boil. Break up the sardines with a fork, reduce the heat, and simmer for 10 minutes. Remove the saucepan from the heat and set it aside.

Coat each tuna steak with a little of the reserved oil. Season the tuna well with salt and pepper. Heat a large nonstick skillet (big enough to hold the fish in 1 layer without packing tightly) over medium-high heat. When the skillet is hot, add the tuna and cook until the bottom browns, about 2 minutes. Quickly turn over the tuna and cook over medium heat for 2 minutes, adding a few tablespoons of water to the pan. (You want to keep the center a little pink, but not sushi-style rare.)

Meanwhile, gently reheat the sauce. Remove the tuna from the skillet and transfer it to 4 large warm plates. Top the tuna with the warm sauce and serve immediately.

Serves 4

nutritionist's note: Read the nutrition labels of jarred marinara sauce and choose one that has 5 or fewer grams of carbohydrates per ½ cup and does not have sugar in its first 5 ingredients.

CTC	Total Carbs	Fiber	Total Fat	Sat Fat	Protein	Calories
4.14	5.14	1.00	14.67	2.20	57.49	396

roasted bluefish with red onions and sage

You don't often associate sage with fish because it's a very powerful herb. But full-flavored bluefish holds its own with both sage and onions. Make sure you buy the fish from a trustworthy fishmonger because bluefish has a short shelf life and needs to be impeccably fresh.

1 center-cut bluefish fillet (3 pounds), with skin
1 large bunch sage
1 pound medium red onions

Preheat the oven to 500°F.

Using a thin-bladed sharp knife, remove the dark oily flesh from the middle of the fish and discard.

Remove the stems from the sage. Fill the channel in the fish (where the dark flesh used to be) with sage leaves, packing them tightly. Save a few sage leaves for garnishing. Season the fish with salt and freshly ground black pepper.

Peel the onions and slice them into very thin rounds. Scatter the onions in the center of a rimmed baking sheet. Place the fish, skin side up, on top of the onions, tucking them under the fish. Add ¼ cup water to the baking sheet.

Roast for 22 to 25 minutes, depending on the thickness of the fish. The skin will become slightly crisp. Turn the fish over onto a cutting board and cut it into 6 portions. Top with the roasted onions. Cut the reserved sage leaves into thin strips and sprinkle over the fish. Serve with any pan juices.

Serves 6

nutritionist's note: Bluefish is considered one of those great "oily" fishes, an excellent source of omega-3 fatty acids.

CTC	Total Carbs	Fiber	Total Fat	Sat Fat	Protein	Calories
5.17	6.60	1.43	9.75	2.10	46.37	310

teriyaki bluefish
with poached scallions

You'll like the vaguely Asian quality of this dish in which the scallions function both as a component of the sauce and as a lovely vegetable. The preparation also works well with salmon, another rich fish.

4	thick bluefish fillets, with skin (8 ounces each)
¾	cup teriyaki sauce
3	large bunches thick scallions (about 8 ounces)

Place the fish in a shallow baking dish. Pour the teriyaki sauce over the fish. Marinate for 30 minutes.

Meanwhile, trim the roots from the scallions. Remove all but 1" of the dark green tops from 2 bunches of scallions and discard the dark green tops. Place the scallions in a skillet with enough salted water just to cover. Bring the water to a boil, then lower the heat and cook until the scallions are soft, about 5 minutes. Remove the skillet from the heat and keep the scallions warm.

Remove the fish from the marinade. Reserve the marinade. Season the skinless side of the fish with coarsely ground black pepper. Heat 1 very large or 2 smaller nonstick skillets until very hot. Put the fish, skin side up, in the skillet and place a large, heavy skillet on top to act as a weight. Cook the fish over medium-high heat for 3 minutes. Turn the fish and cook 3 minutes longer, weighted down again.

Finely dice the remaining bunch of scallions to yield ½ cup. Add the scallions to the reserved marinade. Remove the weight from the fish and add the marinade to the skillet along with ½ cup water. Heat for 1 to 2 minutes, or until the fish is cooked as desired. Serve immediately with the poached scallions that have been quickly warmed in their poaching liquid then thoroughly drained.

Serves 4

CTC	Total Carbs	Fiber	Total Fat	Sat Fat	Protein	Calories
8.72	10.19	1.47	9.72	2.09	49.44	344

vegetables and side dishes

This chapter proves you can eat well, eat happily, eat your vegetables, and maintain a low-carb diet. There are recipes that will nicely complement a steak or chop, and there are recipes that are glorious by themselves as first courses. There are also recipes that, combined, would make a fabulous vegetarian feast.

My herbalist-guru, Dale Glasser Bellisfield, RN, advises "to eat all the colors." Scientists confirm that brightly colored vegetables are loaded with protective phytochemicals that keep the mind and body ticking. Vegetables—the "good" carbs—are chock-a-block with antioxidants that protect the body's cells and bolster our biological defenses.

So no matter what low-carb plan you may be on, it's important to get your carbs from vegetables and fruit, not processed and packaged low-carb foods. In the long run, the key to following any low-carb plan is to keep it interesting. With 41 wonderfully enticing vegetable recipes, this chapter does just that. You will find Snow Peas with Ginger Butter (page 212), Broccoli Smothered in Wine and Olive Oil (page 194), Confit of Carrots and Lemon (page 197), and Slow-Cooked Zucchini with Thyme (page 221).

The mantra, of course, is "fresh, fresh, fresh." That means buying from roadside stands in season or visiting local farmers markets that are springing up around the country, where the happy objective is to lure you with a really ripe tomato.

vegetarian meals

You may have found, as have I, that when entertaining a large crowd, especially around the holidays, there is always at least one guest who prefers veggies to meat or poultry. Rather than prepare special main courses, I usually pass around large platters of various vegetables, family-style, and people help themselves as they wish.

Whether or not you have vegetarians at your table, you can compose eye-catching (and palate-pleasing) arrangements of Roasted Glazed Onions (page 208) alongside Green Beans with Pesto and Walnuts (page 204) or Sugar Snaps with Yellow Pepper Julienne (page 215) alongside a batch of Almond-Crusted Baked Tomatoes (page 216)—colorful, contrasting preparations that hold their own with whatever protein you may (or may not) be serving.

organic produce

I suggest using organic vegetables whenever possible because they just taste better, pure and simple. Once the exclusive domain of health food stores, organic fruits, vegetables, and grains are now available in many chain supermarkets. They are grown without pesticides, so you're doing good for the planet as well as your body.

There are a handful of recipes for starch-based side dishes as well, but none so high in carbs as to exceed our limits. You will find wild rice, whole wheat couscous, bulghur, and white beans, all fitting into the indulgent low-carb (ILC) category.

Also look to the Soups and Starters offerings (beginning on page 69) for more great vegetable ideas, such as Chilled Asparagus with Creamy Sesame Dressing (page 93) and Bibb Lettuce and Roasted Pepper Salad with Creamy Feta Dressing (page 96).

Almost all of the recipes in this chapter are vegetarian, and nearly all are dairy free. Fitting neatly into many healthy eating plans, they only begin to scratch the surface of the beneficent earth.

oven-roasted asparagus with fried capers

If I am famous for one dish, this may be it. Blasting the asparagus in a hot oven keeps them green yet slightly caramelized. Crispy-fried capers add unexpected zing.

2	pounds medium asparagus
¼	cup extra-virgin olive oil
¼	cup large capers in brine, drained

Preheat the oven to 500°F.

Remove the woody bottoms of the asparagus, then trim the stalks to equal lengths. Drizzle 2 tablespoons of the oil on a rimmed baking sheet. Place the asparagus on the baking sheet and toss to coat it with the oil. Lightly sprinkle with salt. Roast the asparagus in the oven for 8 minutes, shaking the pan back and forth once or twice so the vegetables don't stick. When just tender and slightly blackened, transfer the asparagus to a warm platter.

Meanwhile, in a small skillet over medium-high heat, heat the remaining 2 tablespoons oil. Add the capers and fry them, stirring, for 1 minute. Pour the capers and any oil over the asparagus and pass the pepper mill at the table.

Serves 4

nutritionist's note: One-quarter cup of capers has only .5 CTC and no saturated fat. They are a great, almost carb free add-on for many dishes.

CTC	Total Carbs	Fiber	Total Fat	Sat Fat	Protein	Calories
5.10	9.69	4.59	13.98	1.96	4.87	168

poached asparagus with wasabi butter

Celebrate spring by serving this alongside grilled fish, roasted chicken, a thick rare steak . . . you get the idea. Wasabi is a root vegetable from Japan that is similar in flavor to the sharp, bright taste of horseradish. It can be easily found in powdered form in small tins in many supermarkets and most Asian markets.

5	tablespoons unsalted butter, at room temperature
1	tablespoon wasabi powder
2	pounds thick asparagus

Cut the butter into pieces and place it in a bowl. Mix the wasabi powder with ½ tablespoon water to make a paste. Add the paste to the butter with a pinch of salt. Beat the mixture with an electric mixer until the wasabi is incorporated. Scrape the mixture into a ball in the bowl. Refrigerate the mixture until cold.

Remove the woody bottoms of the asparagus, then trim the stalks to equal lengths. With a vegetable peeler and using a light touch, peel the stalks. Fill a 12" sauté pan with 1½" of water. Add salt and bring to a boil. Add the asparagus and cook until the stalks are easily pierced with the tip of a sharp knife, about 10 minutes. They should still be bright green. Drain the asparagus well and place on a platter.

Using a small spoon, scrape curls of the wasabi butter onto the hot asparagus. Sprinkle with salt and coarsely ground black pepper. Serve immediately.

Serves 6

nutritionist's note: Asparagus is perfect for low-carb eating. Six large spears have only 2.93 CTC, and the fiber in them will help keep you feeling full.

CTC	Total Carbs	Fiber	Total Fat	Sat Fat	Protein	Calories
3.45	6.33	2.88	9.87	6.03	3.18	117

steamed broccoli with stir-fried pecans

Chinese oyster sauce, available in the Asian section of most supermarkets and some health food stores, adds a salty, complex flavor to stir-fried broccoli. Read the label of various oyster sauces and choose one that is free of chemical preservatives. You can cut the florets from a large bunch of broccoli or simply buy 1 pound of fresh, precut florets. This recipe is the best way imaginable to get anyone to eat broccoli, but don't reveal the secret ingredient until you get raves.

1   large bunch broccoli (about 1½ pounds)
½   cup coarsely chopped pecans
3   tablespoons Chinese oyster sauce

Cut the broccoli into large florets, leaving 1½" of the stem attached. (You will have about 1 pound florets.) Reserve the remaining stalks for another use. Place the broccoli in a steamer basket and steam over a pot of boiling water, covered, until soft but still bright green, 10 to 12 minutes. Drain well.

Meanwhile, in a small nonstick skillet over medium heat, toast the pecans until they become dark brown, about 1 minute, being careful not to let them burn.

In a large bowl, toss the hot broccoli with the toasted pecans and oyster sauce. Season with freshly ground black pepper. Add salt to taste. (Oyster sauce is salty, so you may not need to add any.) Serve immediately.

Serves 4

CTC	Total Carbs	Fiber	Total Fat	Sat Fat	Protein	Calories
3.49	8.33	4.84	11.11	.98	4.78	136

broccoli smothered in wine and olive oil

Though broccoli is often served bright green and crisp-tender, in this dish it should be soft and yielding, not al dente. Use the best olive oil you can afford.

1	large bunch broccoli (about 1½ pounds)
1	cup Chardonnay
3	tablespoons extra-virgin olive oil

Remove the florets from the broccoli and separate them into large pieces. With a vegetable peeler, peel the stems and slice them into ⅓"-thick rounds.

Bring a 4-quart pot of salted water to a boil. Add the broccoli florets and sliced stems and boil for 8 minutes. Drain the broccoli in a colander, reserving ½ cup cooking liquid. Return the broccoli to the pot with the ½ cup cooking liquid and add the Chardonnay, 2 tablespoons of the oil, ½ teaspoon coarse salt, and ¼ teaspoon whole black peppercorns. Bring to a boil. Cover the pot, reduce the heat to low, and simmer until the broccoli is tender, 20 to 22 minutes.

With a slotted spoon, transfer the broccoli to a shallow bowl or platter. Cook the liquid in the pot over high heat until it is reduced to about ½ cup. Pour over the hot broccoli. Drizzle with the remaining oil, sprinkle with coarse salt, and serve immediately.

Serves 4

CTC	Total Carbs	Fiber	Total Fat	Sat Fat	Protein	Calories
3.78	8.20	4.42	10.64	1.45	4.45	171

brussels sprouts with fresh orange butter

This will make a great addition to your holiday table. All the parts of the orange are used—zest, segments, and juice—to brighten the cabbage-y flavor of Brussels sprouts. Use the smallest sprouts you can find.

1	medium orange
1	pound small Brussels sprouts
3	tablespoons unsalted butter

Grate the zest of the orange and set it aside. Using a small, sharp knife, cut the rind from the orange, removing all of the white pith. Cut the orange between the membranes to release the segments and put them in a bowl. Save any juices that accumulate in a smaller bowl.

Bring a pot of salted water to a boil. Wash and trim the Brussels sprouts, removing any dark outer leaves. Add the Brussels sprouts to the pot and boil for 8 minutes. Drain the Brussels sprouts in a colander.

In a large nonstick skillet over medium heat, melt the butter. Add the Brussels sprouts, orange segments, and zest and cook, stirring, for 5 minutes. Add all of the accumulated juices from the orange, increase the heat to high, and cook for 1 minute longer. Add salt and freshly ground black pepper to taste. Serve immediately.

Serves 4

nutritionist's note: A member of the cruciferous family, Brussels sprouts are full of vitamin C and are a good source of fiber.

CTC	Total Carbs	Fiber	Total Fat	Sat Fat	Protein	Calories
7.75	11.98	4.23	8.95	5.44	3.46	131

savoy cabbage with bacon and cumin

This is a lovely winter vegetable to accompany roast chicken, roast turkey, or even to "winterize" simple grilled fish. Toasted cumin seeds add distinctive flavor and unexpected crunch.

1   large head savoy cabbage (about 1½ pounds)
7   slices nitrite-free bacon
2   tablespoons cumin seeds

Discard the very dark outer leaves of the cabbage. Cut the cabbage in half through the stem end and slice it paper-thin across the width.

Cut the bacon into 1" pieces. In a very large nonstick skillet or a pot large enough to hold all of the cabbage, add the bacon and cook it over medium heat until the fat is rendered and the bacon begins to crisp. Add the cabbage and cook, stirring, until the cabbage begins to wilt, about 10 minutes. Add ½ cup water, coarsely ground black pepper, and salt, if needed. Cook, stirring occasionally, until the water evaporates and the cabbage is tender, about 8 minutes longer.

Meanwhile, in a small skillet over medium heat, toast the cumin seeds with a pinch of salt, stirring constantly, until fragrant and crispy, about 1 minute.

When the cabbage is done, sprinkle with the toasted cumin seeds and serve hot.

Serves 4

CTC	Total Carbs	Fiber	Total Fat	Sat Fat	Protein	Calories
4.30	7.97	3.67	11.21	3.51	9.72	164

confit of carrots and lemon

Carrots do not have to be shunned entirely in a low-carb regime, and this is the most delicious way I know to serve them. The interesting technique, in which carrots are slowly "braised" in a mixture of oil and water, produces a wonderfully tender texture and edible lemon slices. You may substitute bunches of fresh baby carrots or cut larger carrots into a variety of shapes, but don't use those machine-made nubbins that are packaged as "baby carrots."

1½   pounds medium carrots
2   medium lemons
3½   tablespoons extra-virgin olive oil

Peel the carrots and slice on the bias into long ovals ¼" thick. Place the carrots in a 4-quart nonreactive pot with a cover. Halve 1 lemon and squeeze the juice into the pot. Finely slice the remaining lemon and add to the pot. Add the oil, ⅓ cup water, ½ teaspoon coarse salt, and ½ teaspoon whole black peppercorns. Bring the mixture to a boil, then cover the pot and reduce the heat to maintain a simmer. Cook for 35 to 40 minutes without lifting the lid, shaking the pot back and forth several times during the cooking.

Uncover the pot and stir. Add more salt and freshly ground black pepper to taste, if desired, and serve.

Serves 6

CTC	Total Carbs	Fiber	Total Fat	Sat Fat	Protein	Calories
8.04	11.73	3.69	8.11	1.10	1.20	114

roasted cauliflower with cheddar cheese

Roasting small cauliflower florets turns them into yielding, golden nuggets that become addictive, especially when topped with sharp cheddar. Freshly grated Parmesan can be substituted.

1   large head cauliflower
3   tablespoons extra-virgin olive oil
2   ounces sharp white cheddar cheese

Preheat the oven to 425°F.

Remove the core from the cauliflower and discard it. Break the cauliflower into small florets, about ¾" pieces. Place the cauliflower in a bowl, toss with the oil, and sprinkle it with salt and freshly ground black pepper. Place the cauliflower on a rimmed baking sheet and roast for 30 to 45 minutes, until soft and caramelized, turning once during the cooking.

Meanwhile, grate the cheese on the medium holes of a box grater and set it aside.

Transfer the cauliflower to a platter, sprinkle with salt and pepper to taste, and toss. Sprinkle the cauliflower with the cheese. Serve hot or at room temperature.

Serves 4

nutritionist's note: This dish has become a stand-in for "cheese fries" for my vegetable-phobic son, and it is also a good source of vitamin C.

CTC	Total Carbs	Fiber	Total Fat	Sat Fat	Protein	Calories
3.87	7.96	4.09	15.21	4.42	7.30	186

simple fried cauliflower

This is the way my mother made cauliflower at home. The second cooking infuses the cauliflower with the garlic's essence and makes it sweet and user-friendly.

1   large head cauliflower
3   large cloves garlic, sliced paper-thin
⅓   cup extra-virgin olive oil

Remove any leaves and the core from the cauliflower. Cut the cauliflower into small florets, about ½". Bring a medium pot of salted water to a rapid boil. Add the cauliflower and continue to cook over high heat until the cauliflower just becomes tender but is still a bit crisp, 5 to 6 minutes. Drain the cauliflower in a colander under cold running water. Pat the cauliflower dry with paper towels.

In a 12" nonstick skillet over medium heat, heat the garlic and oil. Cook, stirring, until the garlic just turns golden, but not brown, 2 to 3 minutes. Add the cauliflower and cook over high heat, stirring constantly, until the cauliflower browns and starts to look "fried," 10 to 12 minutes. Season with salt and freshly ground white pepper and serve immediately.

Serves 6

CTC	Total Carbs	Fiber	Total Fat	Sat Fat	Protein	Calories
2.92	5.68	2.76	12.26	1.66	2.61	135

braised endive with bay leaves

Most people think of endive as a salad component, but it also makes a tasty and very low-carb cooked vegetable. Braising endives with bay leaves perfumes them in a deliciously subtle way.

6   medium endives
½   cup extra-virgin olive oil
12   fresh bay leaves or dried California bay leaves

Several hours before you plan to serve, remove any dark outer leaves from the endives and discard them. Place the endives in a shallow baking dish with a cover. Pour the oil over the endives. Place the bay leaves under, in between, and on top of the endives. Cover and marinate for several hours at room temperature.

Preheat the oven to 275°F.

Lightly sprinkle the endives with salt. Cover and bake for 1½ hours, shaking several times during the baking. Serve immediately or reheat briefly at 475°F before serving. Add salt and freshly ground black pepper to taste. Decorate with the bay leaves and serve.

Serves 6

nutritionist's note: An entire Belgian endive contains only .5 CTC and so makes a great, crunchy snack and salad toss-in.

CTC	Total Carbs	Fiber	Total Fat	Sat Fat	Protein	Calories
.43	5.70	5.27	18.34	2.51	2.13	188

sautéed escarole with garlic

Here's a thoroughly Italian technique for softening this leafy green's bitter edge. It's excellent served with roast chicken or grilled veal chops.

1	large head escarole (about 1 pound)
2½	tablespoons extra-virgin olive oil
5	large cloves garlic, sliced paper-thin

Remove the core from the escarole. Cut the escarole into 1½" pieces. Wash the escarole well in a colander under cold running water. Dry thoroughly.

In a very large nonstick skillet with a cover, heat the oil over medium heat. Add the garlic and cook until just soft, without browning it at all.

Add the escarole (it will wilt considerably), salt, and freshly ground black pepper. Cook over high heat, stirring constantly, for 1 to 2 minutes. Reduce the heat to medium and cover the skillet. Cook until the escarole is soft but still retains its shape, 10 to 15 minutes. Serve immediately.

Serves 4

CTC	Total Carbs	Fiber	Total Fat	Sat Fat	Protein	Calories
1.96	6.57	4.61	8.80	1.23	2.17	106

asiago-roasted fennel

Slow baking these pale-green bulbs brings out their natural sugars, which are then balanced by the slightly salty cheese crust. Serve this hot as a side dish or at room temperature as part of an antipasto offering.

2   medium-large fennel bulbs, with fronds
¼   cup extra-virgin olive oil
½   cup grated Asiago cheese

Preheat the oven to 400°F.

Trim the fronds and stalks from the fennel bulbs. Set aside the fronds and discard the stalks. Trim any dark spots from the fennel. Cut the bulbs in half lengthwise through the root ends. Place the bulbs, cut sides up, in a shallow baking dish. Rub salt and freshly ground black pepper into the cut sides. Drizzle each half with ½ tablespoon oil. Bake for 25 minutes. Turn the bulbs over, adding a little more oil if necessary. Reduce the heat to 350°F and bake 20 minutes longer. Turn the fennel over again so the cut sides are up. Sprinkle each half with about 2 tablespoons grated cheese and bake for 5 minutes longer. Finely chop some of the reserved fronds, sprinkle over the roasted fennel, and serve.

Serves 6

CTC	Total Carbs	Fiber	Total Fat	Sat Fat	Protein	Calories
3.93	6.65	2.72	11.18	2.49	3.86	137

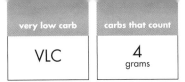

frenched beans with warm vinaigrette

Splitting the beans in half lengthwise makes for a more elegant presentation and provides more surface area for the dressing.

1	pound fresh young green beans
¼	cup extra-virgin olive oil
2	tablespoons red wine vinegar

Trim the ends of the beans. Using a small, sharp knife, cut the beans in half lengthwise to make long, thin halves.

Bring a medium pot of salted water to a boil. Add the beans and cook until tender but still bright green, 3 to 4 minutes. Drain immediately.

In a bowl, whisk together the oil and vinegar and toss with the warm beans. Add coarse salt and freshly ground black pepper to taste and serve.

Serves 4

nutritionist's note: Almost 75 percent of the fat in olive oil is monounsaturated. This helps your heart by lowering bad cholesterol (LDL) while maintaining the good cholesterol (HDL).

CTC	Total Carbs	Fiber	Total Fat	Sat Fat	Protein	Calories
3.82	7.29	3.47	13.62	1.85	1.86	151

green beans with pesto and walnuts

Anyone who loves old-fashioned green beans almondine will love this verdant preparation because it has more crunch and more flavor. It can be served at any temperature, so it can be made ahead.

¾ **pound green beans**
⅓ **cup walnut pieces**
¼ **cup good-quality prepared pesto**

With a small, sharp knife, trim the ends of the beans. Cut the beans in half through the width.

Bring a pot of water, fitted with a steamer basket, to a boil. Place the beans in the steamer basket and cover the pot. Steam until the beans are tender but still bright green, about 6 minutes.

In a small nonstick skillet over medium-high heat, place the walnuts and cook, stirring constantly, until lightly toasted, about 1 minute. Sprinkle lightly with salt and set aside.

When the beans are cooked, shake off any moisture. Put the pesto in a medium-large bowl. Add the beans to the bowl with the pesto and toss quickly. Add salt and freshly ground black pepper to taste. Scatter the toasted nuts over the beans and serve hot or at room temperature.

Serves 4

CTC	Total Carbs	Fiber	Total Fat	Sat Fat	Protein	Calories
4.20	8.07	3.87	9.81	1.12	5.81	133

string beans with roasted garlic butter

The roasted garlic butter, which you make yourself, is also dreamy on steamed broccoli, sugar snaps or snow peas, or atop any sautéed leafy greens. Garlic butter can be made in advance and stored in the fridge for 2 to 3 days.

1   large bulb garlic
¼   cup sweet whipped butter, at room temperature
1   pound green beans or wax beans

Preheat the oven to 400°F.

Wrap the whole bulb of garlic in a pouch of aluminum foil, making sure to tightly crimp the edges all around. Place the garlic in a metal baking pan and roast for 1¼ hours. Remove the garlic from the oven and let cool. Cut in half through the equator and squeeze out the pulp into a medium-large bowl. Add the butter to the bowl and mash together with the garlic pulp. Set aside at room temperature.

Meanwhile, bring a pot of salted water to a boil. Trim the ends of the beans. Add the beans to the boiling water and cook over high heat until the beans are just tender, about 6 minutes. Immediately drain the beans in a colander, shaking off any excess water. Add the beans to the bowl with the garlic butter and toss quickly. Add salt and freshly ground black pepper to taste. Serve immediately.

Serves 4

CTC	Total Carbs	Fiber	Total Fat	Sat Fat	Protein	Calories
6.57	10.58	4.01	7.80	4.78	2.62	114

roasted portobellos on rosemary branches

I've combined three big, highly aromatic components that result in a dish with enough style to be served as a first course or as an accompaniment to something simple like a grilled steak or roast chicken.

1	pound medium portobello mushrooms
¼	cup garlic-flavored olive oil
2	large bunches rosemary

Preheat the oven to 425°F.

Wipe the mushrooms clean with a damp cloth and trim the woody bottoms. Cut the larger mushrooms into quarters and the smaller ones in half. Place the mushrooms in a bowl and pour the oil over the mushrooms. Lightly sprinkle the mushrooms with coarse salt and freshly ground black pepper. Toss well and let sit for 10 minutes.

Remove 1 large sprig rosemary. Scatter the remaining rosemary branches in the center of a rimmed baking sheet to make a large mat for the mushrooms. Place the mushrooms on the rosemary branches. Roast for 12 to 15 minutes, until the mushrooms have just softened. (Do not overcook.)

Finely chop the leaves of the remaining rosemary sprig. Remove the mushrooms from the oven and transfer them to a platter with some of the rosemary branches. Sprinkle the mushrooms with the freshly chopped rosemary. Serve immediately.

Serves 4

CTC	Total Carbs	Fiber	Total Fat	Sat Fat	Protein	Calories
3.29	4.71	1.42	13.90	1.89	3.30	148

shiitake mushrooms in sherry-pepper cream

Yes, it is possible to have a rich creamy dish that is low in calories. This preparation is both a vegetable and a sauce at the same time and goes wonderfully with roast meats or poultry.

10   ounces fresh shiitake mushrooms
½   cup half-and-half
3   tablespoons dry sherry, preferably fino

Wipe the mushrooms clean with a damp cloth and trim off most of the stems. Cut the larger mushrooms in half.

In a medium nonstick skillet over high heat, cook the half-and-half until it starts to thicken and bubble. Add 2 tablespoons of the sherry and the mushrooms. Cook, stirring constantly, until the mushrooms begin to soften, about 3 minutes. Add the remaining tablespoon sherry, salt, and lots of coarsely ground black pepper and cook until the mushrooms give up some of their liquid, 1 to 2 minutes longer. Most of the sauce will be absorbed by the mushrooms.

With a slotted spoon, transfer the mushrooms to a warm shallow bowl. Cook the remaining sauce over high heat, until thickened, and pour over the mushrooms. Serve hot.

Serves 4

CTC	Total Carbs	Fiber	Total Fat	Sat Fat	Protein	Calories
3.56	4.41	.85	3.71	2.19	2.95	69

roasted glazed onions

An hour, more or less, in a hot oven concentrates an onion's inherent sweetness, which is enhanced by the sweet-tart balsamic vinegar. You need only invest about 3 minutes of your time, and you can let the oven do the rest.

3	very large yellow onions
¼	cup extra-virgin olive oil
3	tablespoons balsamic vinegar

Preheat the oven to 425°F.

Peel the onions and halve them through their equators. Put the cut sides down in a heavy shallow baking dish (preferably metal) or on a rimmed baking sheet. Pour 2 tablespoons of the oil over the onions. Add a sprinkling of coarse salt and freshly ground black pepper. Bake for 20 minutes. (The cut sides of the onions will be blackened.) Turn the onions over and flatten them with a spatula. Bake for another 15 minutes. Turn again, flatten with a spatula, and bake for another 20 minutes, until the onions are soft and caramelized.

Remove the onions from the baking dish. Add the remaining 2 tablespoons oil and the vinegar to the pan. Cook over high heat for 1 minute and pour over the onions.

Serves 6

nutritionist's note: Onions can help improve cholesterol levels. Their sulfur compounds help raise your good HDL levels while lowering the dangerous triglycerides.

CTC	Total Carbs	Fiber	Total Fat	Sat Fat	Protein	Calories
6.12	7.47	1.35	9.12	1.23	.87	113

sautéed peas with pancetta and mint

Pancetta, an Italian version of cured bacon, is unsmoked, so it bathes the sweet peas in a rich and slightly porky background flavor. I like to make this all year long because it works well with fresh or frozen peas.

3   cups shelled peas (about 3 pounds pods) or 3 cups frozen peas
3   ounces pancetta
3   tablespoons chopped mint or dill

Bring a saucepan of salted water to a boil. Add the peas and cook until barely tender and still bright green. The cooking time will depend on the size and age of the peas. Drain thoroughly.

Cut the pancetta into ¼" dice. Put the diced pancetta in a medium nonstick skillet and cook over medium heat, stirring often, until the pancetta renders some of its fat and begins to get a little crispy. Add the peas and cook, stirring frequently, until softened, adding a few tablespoons of water if necessary. Add salt and freshly ground black pepper to taste. Quickly stir in the mint or dill and serve.

Serves 6

CTC	Total Carbs	Fiber	Total Fat	Sat Fat	Protein	Calories
6.10	9.19	3.09	6.46	2.03	7.86	124

rainbow pepper confit

Here "confit" means slow cooking in a covered pan in oil and vinegar—half braising, half steaming—until the peppers become incredibly sweet and tender. It's a simple technique that works well with many vegetables. This colorful dish can be used as a condiment atop a juicy rare burger or grilled fish, or alongside a simple omelet.

4   medium-large bell peppers (red, yellow, orange, or a combination)
¼   cup extra-virgin olive oil
2   tablespoons or more Spanish sherry vinegar

Wash and dry the peppers. Cut each pepper in half lengthwise. Remove the core and any seeds. Cut each half into 5 long strips.

In a heavy medium pot with a cover, add the pepper strips, oil, 2 tablespoons vinegar, and ½ teaspoon whole black peppercorns. Bring to a boil. Cover the pot, reduce the heat, and simmer for 45 minutes without lifting the cover. (The steam helps soften the peppers.) Shake the pot back and forth several times during the cooking.

Transfer the peppers and juices to a platter. Add salt to taste and sprinkle with additional vinegar. Serve warm, at room temperature, or chilled.

Serves 4

CTC	Total Carbs	Fiber	Total Fat	Sat Fat	Protein	Calories
7.42	10.54	3.12	13.81	1.87	1.46	166

roasted peppers with balsamic syrup and toasted pine nuts

These 3 ingredients harmonize incredibly well and are a robust accompaniment to steak or grilled chicken. This recipe also can be an enticing first course. It's best served slightly warm or at room temperature.

4   large red bell peppers
¼   cup pine nuts
6   tablespoons balsamic vinegar

Preheat the broiler.

Place the peppers on a baking sheet and broil, about 6" from the heat, for several minutes on all sides, until completely blackened. Transfer the peppers to a paper bag, close tightly, and let steam for 5 to 10 minutes to loosen the skin. Or you can put the blackened peppers in a bowl and place a large plate on top to fit tightly so that no steam will escape. Let sit for 5 to 10 minutes.

Meanwhile, in a small nonstick skillet over medium heat, toast the pine nuts, stirring constantly, until golden, about 1 minute.

Remove the peppers from the bag or bowl and scrape off all the blackened skin. (Do not rinse the peppers.) Cut the peppers, lengthwise, into quarters, removing the core and seeds. Arrange on a platter to collect any juices. Sprinkle the peppers lightly with salt and let cool.

In a small nonstick skillet, bring the vinegar to a boil. Cook over high heat for a few minutes until reduced by half. Let cool, then drizzle over the peppers. Add a dusting of freshly ground black pepper and scatter the pine nuts on top.

Serves 6

CTC	Total Carbs	Fiber	Total Fat	Sat Fat	Protein	Calories
7.41	9.85	2.44	3.11	.48	2.35	72

snow peas with ginger butter

Fresh ginger and snow peas combine here in an elegant Asian-inspired side dish that cohabits nicely with almost any fish preparation.

1   pound snow peas
2   tablespoons unsalted butter
1   4" piece fresh ginger

Using a small, sharp knife, trim the ends of the snow peas. Remove the string running down the side of each snow pea.

Bring a pot of water, fitted with a steamer basket, to a boil. Put the snow peas in the steamer basket and cover. Steam until the snow peas are crisp-tender but still bright green, about 8 minutes.

Meanwhile, put the butter in a medium-large bowl. Using a small, sharp knife, peel the ginger. Grate the ginger on the large holes of a box grater. Put the pulp in a paper towel and squeeze the juice into the bowl with the butter. Thoroughly blend the juice into the butter. Discard the grated ginger.

Remove the snow peas from the steamer, shaking off any excess water. Add the snow peas to the bowl and toss until the snow peas are coated with butter. Add salt to taste. Serve immediately.

Serves 4

CTC	Total Carbs	Fiber	Total Fat	Sat Fat	Protein	Calories
7.07	10.13	3.06	5.78	3.59	2.69	96

stir-fried spinach with sesame seeds

The curly spinach called for here has more flavor than flat and smaller baby spinach, which is more appropriate for salads. Feel free to use regular spinach if curly is not available. I've added sesame seeds for an interesting textural boost.

2   pounds curly spinach
2½ tablespoons garlic-flavored olive oil
1   tablespoon toasted sesame seeds

Remove any tough stems from the spinach and discard. If the spinach is not prewashed, thoroughly wash the leaves in a colander. Drain well and spin dry in a salad spinner.

In a large wok or a very large nonstick skillet over medium-high heat, heat 2 tablespoons of the oil. Add the spinach and toss just until it wilts and softens. (Do not overcook because you want the spinach to stay bright green.) Remove the spinach from the heat, add salt and freshly ground black pepper to taste, and toss. Drizzle with the remaining ½ tablespoon oil. Sprinkle with the sesame seeds and serve immediately.

Serves 4

nutritionist's note: Sesame seeds are high in healthy fats and have only 1.3 CTC per tablespoon.

CTC	Total Carbs	Fiber	Total Fat	Sat Fat	Protein	Calories
1.96	8.07	6.11	10.85	1.49	6.44	140

"creamed" spinach

Here is a recipe where frozen spinach works especially well. There is no cream is this dish, but there is a great creamy texture from the pureed cottage cheese and a little butter. This combination is a magical stand-in for the real thing, which is very high in saturated fat, calories, and carbs.

2   packages (10 ounces each) frozen leaf spinach (do not thaw)
1¼   cups low-fat cottage cheese
2½   tablespoons unsalted butter

In a large saucepan with a cover, combine ½ cup water and ½ teaspoon salt and bring to a boil. Add the frozen spinach and bring to a boil. Cover and reduce the heat to medium-high. Cook, stirring several times, for 10 minutes. Drain thoroughly in a colander, being sure to shake out all of the water. Pat spinach dry with paper towels.

Transfer the hot spinach to a food processor. Add the cottage cheese and all but 1 teaspoon of the butter. Process until very, very smooth. Return to the saucepan. Add salt and ground white pepper to taste. Heat gently and transfer to a warm bowl. Place the remaining butter on top and serve.

Serves 4

nutritionist's note: This healthy version saves you a whopping 15 CTC over frozen creamed spinach.

CTC	Total Carbs	Fiber	Total Fat	Sat Fat	Protein	Calories
3.35	7.61	4.26	8.36	5.01	12.97	149

sugar snaps with yellow pepper julienne

This dish is also very beautiful when made with red peppers and is especially festive for the Christmas holidays. It's delicious hot, cold, or in between. Roasted peanut oil can be found in many supermarkets as well as Asian and health food stores. Other flavorful oils—such as walnut oil—can be substituted.

1   pound sugar snap peas
2   medium yellow bell peppers
3   tablespoons roasted peanut oil

Remove the ends of the pea pods and their fibrous strings. Bring a pot of salted water to a boil. Add the peas and boil until they just begin to soften but are still bright green, about 3 minutes. Drain in a colander under cold running water. Pat dry with paper towels.

Cut the peppers in half lengthwise. Remove the core and seeds. Cut 2 of the halves into long, thin strips.

Cut the remaining 2 pepper halves into ½" squares. Place the pepper squares in a blender with 1 tablespoon of the peanut oil, 1 tablespoon water, and a pinch of salt. Process for several minutes, until very smooth.

In a large nonstick skillet over medium heat, heat the remaining 2 tablespoons peanut oil. Add the pepper strips and cook, stirring, until they begin to soften, about 2 minutes. Add the peas and continue cooking, stirring, until just tender, about 2 minutes. Add the yellow pepper sauce, stir, and continue cooking until the mixture is hot, about 3 minutes longer. Add salt and freshly ground black pepper to taste. Serve hot, warm, or room temperature.

Serves 6

nutritionist's note: Don't let "sugar" in the name deter you. Sugar snap peas are fine for a low-carb diet, with only 2 CTC per cooked ½-cup serving.

CTC	Total Carbs	Fiber	Total Fat	Sat Fat	Protein	Calories
5.59	9.25	3.66	6.83	1.15	2.27	104

almond-crusted baked tomatoes

Ground-up almonds and cheese form a flavorful crust for baked tomatoes, which are a time-honored restaurant accompaniment to many main courses. (Restaurants use bread crumbs, though—this is better.)

6	medium-large ripe tomatoes
½	cup sliced almonds, with skins
¾	cup freshly grated Parmesan cheese

Preheat the oven to 425°F.

Cut the stem ends off the tomatoes and scoop out ½" tomato flesh. Salt the insides of the tomatoes and turn them upside down on paper towels to drain.

In a small nonstick skillet over medium heat, toast the almonds, tossing occasionally, until golden, about 1 to 2 minutes. Let cool for 5 minutes. Transfer the almonds to a food processor and process until finely ground. Add the cheese and freshly ground black pepper and pulse to mix.

Fill the tomato cavities with the almond-cheese mixture, mounding it on top. Place the tomatoes on a rimmed baking sheet with a few tablespoons of water. Bake for about 15 minutes, or until the tomatoes are soft and the stuffing is crusted. Serve immediately.

Serves 6

nutritionist's note: Nutrient-dense tomatoes provide lycopene and vitamin C, and almonds are a source of heart-healthy fats.

CTC	Total Carbs	Fiber	Total Fat	Sat Fat	Protein	Calories
6.08	8.59	2.51	7.48	2.28	7.06	122

short-stack tomatoes and onions

This layered, napoleon-like vegetable dish gains intensity from its extended time in the oven. Depending on what else you're serving, you may use a flavored oil—such as basil, chili, or rosemary— for an added flavor dimension.

4   ripe medium tomatoes
2   medium red onions
¼   cup olive oil

Preheat the oven to 375°F.

Using a sharp knife, cut a ¼" slice off the top and bottom of each tomato and discard. Slice each tomato into 3 thick slices and reassemble each to look like a whole tomato.

Peel the onions and slice into eight ¼" slices and 4 thinner slices. Layer the thicker onion slices between the tomato slices, ending with a thin slice of onion on top of each tomato stack. Drizzle 1 tablespoon of the oil over each stack and sprinkle with salt and freshly ground black pepper. Place a short skewer in the center of each stack to help hold them together.

Place the stacks on a rimmed baking sheet and bake for 1¼ hours. Baste with the pan juices twice during the baking, making sure the tomatoes hold their shape. Remove the tomatoes from the oven and let rest 15 minutes. The bottoms will be soft, so use a spatula to carefully transfer them to plates. Spoon the pan juices over the tomatoes and serve.

Serves 4

nutritionist's note: The vitamin C in tomatoes is found in the gel around the seeds. Vine-ripened tomatoes have twice the amount of vitamin C as hothouse types.

CTC	Total Carbs	Fiber	Total Fat	Sat Fat	Protein	Calories
8.11	10.45	2.34	13.99	1.89	1.68	166

sautéed grape tomatoes with shallots

I love the color and texture of these slightly cooked tomatoes and use this recipe whenever a dish needs a visual pick-me-up. Grape tomatoes, which are generally smaller and sweeter than cherry tomatoes, have thicker skins and hold up better during cooking.

3   ounces shallots

2   tablespoons extra-virgin olive oil

12   ounces grape tomatoes

Peel the shallots and finely chop them; you will have about ¼ heaping cup.

In a large nonstick skillet over medium-low heat, heat the oil. Add the shallots and cook, stirring, until just soft, about 3 minutes. Add the tomatoes and cook over high heat, stirring frequently, for about 6 minutes. Do not let the shallots blacken, but they will caramelize slightly. The tomatoes will wilt and get "wrinkled," and that's just what you want. Add salt and freshly ground black pepper to taste and serve.

Serves 4

nutritionist's note: High in vitamin C and antioxidants, four grape tomatoes contain only 1 CTC. Think of them as "nature's candy."

CTC	Total Carbs	Fiber	Total Fat	Sat Fat	Protein	Calories
6.58	7.52	.94	7.05	.95	1.25	93

spaghetti squash, "spaghetti-style"

After eating this dish, my son, who eats a lot of carb-laden pasta, opined that spaghetti squash is an equally good conveyance for marinara sauce. The dish is more nutritious as well.

1	spaghetti squash (2¼ pounds)
¾	cup good-quality marinara sauce
3	ounces sharp provolone cheese, in 1 piece

Preheat the oven to 400°F.

Carefully cut the squash in half lengthwise. (I remove the seeds after cooking since it's easier, but you can scrape them out before cooking if you wish.) Place the squash, cut sides down, on a rimmed baking sheet and pour ½ cup water over the squash. Bake for 50 to 55 minutes, until the squash can be easily pierced with a skewer. (The squash will be soft but still retain its shape.)

Meanwhile, grate the cheese on the medium holes of a box grater and set aside.

A few minutes before removing the squash from the oven, heat the marinara sauce in a small pan until very hot.

Remove the squash from the oven. Scrape out the seeds if need be and discard. Using the tines of a large fork, scrape the flesh of the squash and remove the squash in long threads. Place in 4 medium bowls. Top with hot marinara sauce and sprinkle with cheese. Serve immediately.

Serves 4

nutritionist's note: By switching from spaghetti to spaghetti squash, you get a hearty dose of vitamin A and save over 40 CTC.

CTC	Total Carbs	Fiber	Total Fat	Sat Fat	Protein	Calories
9.44	11.82	2.38	6.93	3.84	6.87	133

roasted spiced acorn squash

So easy to prepare and so savory, this is a perfect fall and winter staple. It also makes the ultimate Thanksgiving vegetable, replacing higher-carb sweet potatoes. Because I've used pumpkin pie spice here, you won't miss the no-no pie for dessert.

2   acorn squashes (1 pound each)
3   tablespoons unsalted butter
2   tablespoons pumpkin pie spice

Preheat the oven to 400°F.

Cut the squashes in half through the root ends. Scoop out the seeds. Place the squash cut sides down on a rimmed baking sheet. Pour ½ cup water over the squash and place in the oven. Bake for 45 minutes, until the squash can be easily pierced with the tip of a knife. Remove from the oven.

Preheat the broiler.

Melt the butter in a small saucepan and, using a pastry brush, brush the insides and tops of the squash with butter. Sprinkle the squash very lightly with salt and freshly ground black pepper, then sprinkle more liberally with the pumpkin pie spice. Place the squash under the broiler, about 6" from the heat, for 30 seconds, until golden. Serve immediately.

Serves 4

nutritionist's note: Winter squashes such as acorn and butternut have higher CTCs than some vegetables, but their high content of vitamin C and beta-carotene make them worth eating.

CTC	Total Carbs	Fiber	Total Fat	Sat Fat	Protein	Calories
11.51	13.59	2.08	9.07	5.57	1.14	130

slow-cooked zucchini with thyme

I happened upon this cooking technique at a restaurant in Rome a few years ago, where they also cooked some small shrimp along with the zucchini. The recipe only works with small zucchini because larger ones contain too much moisture.

6   small zucchini (about 1½ pounds)
1   large bunch thyme
¼   cup extra-virgin olive oil

Cut the zucchini into ¼"-thick rounds. Remove about 3 tablespoons thyme leaves, set aside, and reserve several thyme sprigs for garnish.

In each of 2 large nonstick skillets over low heat, heat 2 tablespoons oil. Place the zucchini in the skillets in 1 layer. Cook slowly until the zucchini are golden on the bottom, about 10 minutes. Carefully turn the zucchini over and cook for 10 minutes on the other side.

To each skillet, add ¼ cup boiling water and a large pinch of salt. Simmer slowly until all of the water has evaporated and the zucchini are soft but still hold their shape, 5 to 10 minutes. Remove the zucchini to a platter and cover to keep warm.

Transfer the oil from one of the skillets to the other. Add the reserved thyme leaves to the skillet with the oil and cook, stirring, until the thyme begins to crisp, about 1 minute. Scatter the thyme leaves and oil over the zucchini and garnish with the reserved thyme sprigs. Add freshly ground black pepper and serve immediately.

Serves 4

nutritionist's note: Do not peel the skin of the zucchini because that's where all the good fiber is. Half a cup of cooked zucchini has only 2.3 CTC, is fat free, and has less than 15 calories.

CTC	Total Carbs	Fiber	Total Fat	Sat Fat	Protein	Calories
3.07	5.37	2.30	13.77	1.88	2.07	145

chilled asparagus with asian dressing

It's the roasted peanut oil that provides the Asian overtones in this unusual asparagus dish, so check the label carefully to make sure that it's roasted, not plain, peanut oil. Dark Asian sesame oil, which has a more pronounced flavor, makes a good substitute. I like this recipe because you can make it ahead of time. It can be served with both hot and cold main courses or from a big bowl at a picnic.

1	pound medium asparagus
3	tablespoons roasted peanut oil
1	tablespoon balsamic vinegar

Remove the woody bottoms of the asparagus, then trim the stalks evenly. With a vegetable peeler, using a light touch, peel the stalks.

Fill a 12" sauté pan with several inches of water. Add salt and bring to a boil. Add the asparagus and cook until the stalks are easily pierced with the tip of a sharp knife, about 8 minutes. (They should still be bright green and crisp-tender.) Drain well under cold water and pat dry with paper towels.

In a small bowl, whisk together the oil and vinegar until emulsified. Add salt and freshly ground black pepper to taste. Pour the dressing over the asparagus and chill until cold before serving.

Serves 4

CTC	Total Carbs	Fiber	Total Fat	Sat Fat	Protein	Calories
3.25	5.65	2.40	10.35	1.78	2.59	118

turkish-style cucumber salad

This is a variation of a Turkish cucumber recipe called cacik. *A little dark sesame oil goes a long way in providing flavor.*

2   medium cucumbers
2   teaspoons dark Asian sesame oil
1   cup low-fat plain yogurt

Peel the cucumbers. Cut the cucumbers in half lengthwise and, using a small spoon, remove the seeds. Slice into ¼"-thick "half-moons." Place in a bowl. Add the oil, yogurt, salt, and freshly ground black pepper. Stir and refrigerate for 1 to 2 hours before serving.

Serves 4

CTC	Total Carbs	Fiber	Total Fat	Sat Fat	Protein	Calories
6.72	7.62	.90	3.27	.86	3.78	72

cucumber salad with mint

This is an incredibly refreshing salad—perfect for a picnic—that provides a lot of fiber for its tiny caloric content. I've used rice vinegar because it is less acidic and more interesting than distilled white vinegar. Do not substitute seasoned rice vinegar.

6   kirby cucumbers (about 1 pound)

⅓   cup Asian rice vinegar (not sweetened)

¼   cup chopped fresh mint, peppermint, or spearmint

Peel the cucumbers. Slice half of them paper-thin and cut the remaining cucumbers into ¼" cubes. In a bowl, toss all of the cucumbers with the vinegar and mint. Season with salt and ground white pepper to taste. Refrigerate for 1 to 2 hours before serving.

Serves 4

CTC	Total Carbs	Fiber	Total Fat	Sat Fat	Protein	Calories
2.88	3.92	1.04	.16	.04	.84	25

cabbage slaw

This is an old-fashioned salad once known as "cream slaw" and is a healthy alternative to the store-bought version.

1	small head green cabbage (about 1¼ pounds)
½	cup heavy cream
3	tablespoons cider vinegar

Very thinly shred the cabbage with a sharp knife. Transfer to a colander in the sink and sprinkle with 1 tablespoon coarse salt. Add a weight on top, such as a heavy pot filled with water. Let sit for 30 minutes. Rinse the cabbage well under cold running water. Dry the cabbage thoroughly with paper towels or spin in a salad spinner.

Put the cabbage in a bowl, pour the cream over it, and mix well. Add the vinegar and freshly ground black pepper and toss well. Refrigerate for 1 hour. Add salt to taste and toss again before serving.

Serves 6

nutritionist's note: Even with the addition of heavy cream, this recipe saves you 27 CTC and 200 calories per serving over store-bought coleslaw.

CTC	Total Carbs	Fiber	Total Fat	Sat Fat	Protein	Calories
4.72	7.46	2.74	7.72	4.65	2.12	100

truffled white bean puree

If you are longing for an ultra-creamy, rich substitute for "forbidden" mashed potatoes, then here it is. Try serving it next to a simply grilled steak or underneath freshly roasted chicken where it will absorb all of the desirable juices. White truffle oil is essential to this dish and worth the splurge. It can be found in specialty food stores and many supermarkets.

½   **pound dried small white beans**
¼   **cup heavy cream**
2   **tablespoons white truffle oil**

Place the beans in a medium pot with enough water to cover by 1". Bring the water to a boil and continue to boil for 2 minutes. Remove from the heat. Cover the pot and let it sit for 1 hour.

Drain the beans in a colander. Transfer the beans to a pot with 12 whole black peppercorns and add enough water to cover by 2". Bring the water to a boil, then reduce the heat, cover, and simmer until the beans are tender, about 1 hour and 20 minutes.

Drain the beans, reserving ½ cup cooking liquid. Transfer the beans to a food processor and process until smooth, adding some of the reserved cooking liquid if necessary. With the motor running, slowly add the cream and truffle oil. Add salt and freshly ground white pepper to taste and mix. Transfer to a small saucepan and gently heat. Serve immediately.

Serves 6

nutritionist's note: Beans should be included in your low-carb lifestyle. They're high in soluble fiber, which helps to lower cholesterol, and have been shown to regulate blood sugar.

CTC	Total Carbs	Fiber	Total Fat	Sat Fat	Protein	Calories
17.31	23.06	5.75	8.52	2.99	9.04	199

wild rice with walnut oil and scallions

Wild rice is actually not rice, but an aquatic grass. Although the portion is modest to keep the carbs in check, its virtues include great flavor, low calories, and almost no saturated fat. It will make a great addition to your holiday table.

1	cup uncooked wild rice
1	bunch scallions
2	tablespoons walnut oil

In a large saucepan with a cover, bring 6 cups salted water to a boil.

In a sieve, wash the rice and add to the boiling water. Reduce the heat, cover, and cook until the rice is tender, 50 to 55 minutes. (The time will vary depending on the type and age of the rice.)

Meanwhile, trim all but 2" of the green tops from the scallions and set the tops aside. Trim the roots from the scallion bottoms. Cut the scallions in half lengthwise, then across into ¼" pieces. (You will have a heaping ¼ cup chopped scallions.)

In a small nonstick skillet over low heat, heat the oil. Add the chopped scallions and cook, stirring occasionally, until very soft but not browned, about 15 minutes. Set aside.

Drain the cooked rice in a colander and transfer to a warm bowl. Add the cooked scallions to the rice and toss quickly. Add salt and a generous amount of freshly ground black pepper. Finely chop the reserved green tops of the scallions to make ¼ cup, sprinkle on the rice, and serve immediately.

Serves 8

nutritionist's note: Wild rice has a much lower glycemic index than white rice, making it a perfect side dish to satisfy any starch cravings.

CTC	Total Carbs	Fiber	Total Fat	Sat Fat	Protein	Calories
14.59	16.29	1.70	3.65	.35	3.26	107

aromatic ginger rice

This wonderful accompaniment is allowable on your plan if you use brown rice and keep the portions small. Use brown basmati rice for maximum flavor.

1   5" piece fresh ginger
1   cup uncooked brown rice
2   tablespoons unsalted butter

Peel the ginger and mince enough of it to get 1 tablespoon. Grate the remaining ginger on the large holes of a box grater. Place the grated ginger in a paper towel and squeeze the juice into a small dish to get about 2 teaspoons fresh ginger juice.

In a medium saucepan, bring 2½ cups water and 1 teaspoon salt to a boil. Add the rice and the minced ginger. Cover, reduce the heat, and simmer until the water has evaporated and the rice is tender, about 20 minutes. Cut the butter into small pieces and stir into the hot rice. Add the ginger juice and salt and ground white pepper to taste. Serve immediately.

Serves 8

nutritionist's note: Do not use instant or parboiled brown rice, which have a higher glycemic index than raw brown rice.

CTC	Total Carbs	Fiber	Total Fat	Sat Fat	Protein	Calories
17.16	17.98	.82	3.56	1.93	1.88	112

bulghur wheat and caramelized shallots

Bulghur, or cracked wheat, is generally used for making tabbouleh and is also great as a hot side dish. It can be found in Middle Eastern markets and health food stores. Be sure to use coarse, not fine, bulghur for this dish. Do not buy packaged, seasoned bulghur either. Lots of caramelized shallots give sweetness and depth of flavor here.

6   ounces shallots (about 8 large cloves)
3   tablespoons olive oil
1   cup coarse bulghur wheat

Peel the shallots and chop coarsely. In a large nonstick skillet over medium-low heat, heat 2 tablespoons of the oil. Add the chopped shallots and cook, stirring occasionally, until dark golden brown, soft, and caramelized, about 20 minutes.

Meanwhile, in a medium bowl, place the bulghur and cover with 2½ cups boiling water. Cover the bowl and let the bulghur sit until softened, about 20 minutes. Drain the excess water, if necessary.

Add the drained bulghur to the cooked shallots in the skillet and cook, stirring frequently, until the bulghur is soft and rather dry, about 10 minutes longer. Add the remaining 1 tablespoon oil, salt, and freshly ground black pepper. Fluff the bulghur with a fork. Serve immediately or gently reheat.

Serves 6

nutritionist's note: Bulghur is a great alternative to rice and is high in fiber and low on the glycemic index.

CTC	Total Carbs	Fiber	Total Fat	Sat Fat	Protein	Calories
16.85	22.02	5.17	7.14	.98	3.45	158

parmesan couscous with toasted pine nuts

Whole wheat couscous is available in health food stores and Middle Eastern markets and makes a trendy, fluffy alternative to rice. It is a great sidekick to many meat and poultry dishes because it absorbs juices like a sponge.

2½ tablespoons pine nuts
1   cup whole wheat couscous
6   tablespoons freshly grated Parmesan cheese

In a small nonstick skillet over medium-high heat, cook the pine nuts, stirring constantly with a wooden spoon, until the nuts turn golden brown, about 1 minute. (Be careful not to overcook because they burn quickly.) Immediately transfer them to a small plate to stop the cooking.

In a small saucepan with a cover, bring 1½ cups salted water to a boil, then reduce the heat to medium-low. Add the couscous and cook, stirring constantly, until the liquid is absorbed but the couscous is still moist, 2 to 3 minutes. Remove from the heat. Cover the saucepan and let sit for 5 minutes.

Fluff the couscous with a fork and transfer to a large warm bowl. Stir in 4 tablespoons of the cheese and the toasted pine nuts. Add salt and freshly ground black pepper to taste, scatter the remaining cheese on top, and serve immediately.

Serves 8

nutritionist's note: Whole wheat couscous, like bulghur, is another great way to get your family to switch to lower glycemic foods and fill them up with satisfaction.

CTC	Total Carbs	Fiber	Total Fat	Sat Fat	Protein	Calories
14.26	17.01	2.75	2.76	.86	5.06	113

whole wheat cumin couscous

The real surprise in this—one of my favorite side dishes—is the chicken fat! A little bit goes a long way in adding great flavor and rich texture. The deeper flavor of whole wheat couscous stands up well against the heady aroma of the toasted cumin. You can buy rendered chicken fat in the poultry section of many supermarkets.

1   tablespoon cumin seeds
1   cup whole wheat couscous
2   tablespoons chicken fat or unsalted butter, at room temperature

In a small nonstick skillet over medium-high heat, cook the cumin seeds, stirring constantly, until the seeds are toasted and crispy, 2 to 3 minutes. Set aside.

In a small saucepan with a cover, place 1½ cups salted water. Add 1 teaspoon of the toasted cumin seeds and bring to a boil. Reduce the heat and add the couscous. Stir until the liquid is absorbed but the couscous is still moist, 2 to 3 minutes. Remove from the heat. Cover the saucepan and let sit for 3 minutes.

Fluff the couscous with a fork and add salt and freshly ground black pepper to taste. Transfer to a warm bowl and add chicken fat or butter and stir until incorporated. Sprinkle with the remaining 2 teaspoons toasted cumin seeds. Serve immediately or gently reheat.

Serves 8

nutritionist's note: Chicken fat has half the saturated fat of butter. You can try it in other recipes to reduce the sat fat and add another layer of flavor.

CTC	Total Carbs	Fiber	Total Fat	Sat Fat	Protein	Calories
13.95	16.59	2.64	3.62	.95	3.04	112

desserts

Nowhere is the expression "the proof of the pudding is in the eating" more apt than with 3-ingredient dessert recipes that are also low carb! The good news is, you can have it all—scrumptious desserts that are remarkably healthy and a cinch to make.

For my own cooking at home, I use sugar in moderation. However, I respect the needs and passions of those who truly cannot have white sugar because of medical issues such as diabetes and of those who are religiously counting carbs as a temporary measure in their lives. But without something sweet, a low-carb lifestyle is hard to sustain.

So I experimented, and experimented, and eventually came to understand how to make desserts using a minimum of sugar substitute (more about that later) or one other artificial sweetener—a low-cal/sugar-free maple-flavored syrup from Maple Grove Farms of Vermont.

The results were serendipitous ... and delicious. For example, there's a strawberry dessert that tastes like cheesecake; peaches that marinate in a red wine–Splenda mixture wind up tasting like the effervescent Italian wine lambrusco; and tahini mixed into melted bittersweet chocolate tastes like a luxurious candy bar.

I used my friends as taste-testers to make sure that these desserts got their blessings. Many of my 3-ingredient recipes that tasted fantastic with real sugar ended up in the trash can when a sugar substitute was used. Some of the tasters had sensitivities to all artificial sweeteners, while others accepted Splenda over other substitutes. And some friends had become so used to artificial sweeteners that they actually liked them better than sugar. It was quite an education.

Thankfully, I am delighted with the offerings that follow. I know they will satisfy thousands of pleasure-seekers who crave sweetness at the end of a meal and who look forward to a sweet snack during the day. Most of these desserts rely on fresh fruits, which we are all encouraged to eat more of, with some refreshing sorbets, ice creams, and several chocolate surprises, too.

As a bonus, almost all of the desserts are very low in calories and low in fat.

In the end, I used Splenda instead of any other sugar substitute in the recipes. Splenda is heat stable so it holds up during cooking. Another popular sweetener, aspartame, is marketed as Equal Spoonfuls and measures cup for cup with real sugar, too. But it is not heat stable and is useful only for cold or uncooked items.

But—there's always a "but"—anything artificial requires some explanation. Do not be misled by Splenda's, or other brands', claims to be free of calories and carbs. Helen Kimmel offers this warning: The FDA says something with less than 1 calorie *per serving* can be labeled as calorie free, and Splenda does indeed have less than 1 calorie per serving—which is 1 teaspoon—but not 0 calories. And most of us use more than 1 teaspoon at a time. The fact is, Splenda has 24 grams of carbohydrates and 96 calories per cup. A cup of Equal Spoonfuls has 23 grams of carbs and 92 calories per cup. Our recipes take these numbers into account.

Stay away from any products that use sugar alcohols like maltitol and sorbitol, which are controversial ingredients. For example, when choosing a maple syrup substitute among the many lining supermarket shelves, select one that is sweetened with Splenda only—not with maltitol or sorbitol.

Splenda, Splenda-sweetened maple syrup substitute, and light whipped topping (without any trans fats) are the only "processed foods" that I allow in this chapter. I have tried all kinds of low-carb syrups and flavorings and other sugar-free substitutes and found them objectionable, including most low-carb processed desserts that were on the market when this chapter was drafted. In truth, these convenience products establish an extremely strong case for making your own yummy treats—from scratch—at home.

In addition to the 24 sweet offerings in this chapter, some may opt for fruit and cheese (see the opposite page for some great ideas) to end their meals, instead of a more traditional sweet.

For the best results, keep it real, keep it simple, and you will reap great satisfaction.

Coffee, anyone?

fruit and cheese and nuts

This is my idea of an immensely satisfying dessert. Fruit, provided it's ripe and flavorful, is a wonderful counterpoint for cheese and lightly toasted nuts. It's a fresh, natural way to end a meal or to enjoy as a healthy snack during the day. Feel free to come up with your own pairings. Here are 6 great ideas to get you started. All make a single serving and are easily multiplied.

apples with cheddar and macadamia nuts

low carb	carbs that count
LC	8 grams

½ small apple
1 ounce low-fat Vermont cheddar cheese
5 small macadamia nuts

Serves 1

nutritionist's note: This trio is a nutritional powerhouse, with soluble fiber from the apple, monounsaturated fat from the macadamia nuts, and protein and calcium from the cheese.

CTC	7.87	Sat Fat	2.96
Total Carbs	10.44	Protein	8.11
Fiber	2.57	Calories	182
Total Fat	12.96		

comice pears with parmesan and almonds

low carb	carbs that count
LC	10 grams

½ small pear
1 ounce Parmesan cheese, preferably real Parmigiano-Reggiano, thinly sliced
4 whole almonds, with skins

Serves 1

nutritionist's note: Pears are a source of boron, a mineral that helps keep your bones and memory strong.

CTC	10.07	Sat Fat	5.61
Total Carbs	12.51	Protein	13.07
Fiber	2.44	Calories	198
Total Fat	11.22		

red grapes with blue cheese and walnuts

low carb	carbs that count
LC	8 grams

8 dark grapes
¾ ounce blue cheese
7 walnut halves

Serves 1

nutritionist's note: The resveratrol in the dark grapes and the omega-3 fatty acids in the walnuts make this a heart-healthy snack.

CTC	8.19	Sat Fat	4.91
Total Carbs	9.54	Protein	6.97
Fiber	1.35	Calories	196
Total Fat	15.59		

fresh cherries with brie and hazelnuts

low carb	carbs that count
LC	7 grams

6 cherries, with stems
¾ ounce ripe brie cheese
10 hazelnuts (about ½ ounce), lightly toasted

Serves 1

CTC	6.9	Sat Fat	4.42
Total Carbs	9.21	Protein	7.02
Fiber	2.31	Calories	189
Total Fat	14.89		

fresh figs with gorgonzola and pine nuts

indulgent low carb	carbs that count
ILC	12.5 grams

2 small fresh ripe figs
1 ounce imported Gorgonzola cheese
1 tablespoon pine nuts, lightly toasted

Serves 1

nutritionist's note: Figs are high in fiber and potassium. In season, they are a wonderful change of pace from everyday fruit.

CTC	12.61	Sat Fat	6.01
Total Carbs	15.31	Protein	8.66
Fiber	2.70	Calories	200
Total Fat	12.72		

peaches with goat cheese and toasted pecans

very low carb	carbs that count
VLC	5 grams

½ ripe medium peach, thinly sliced
1 ounce fresh goat cheese (chèvre)
10 pecan halves, lightly toasted

Serves 1

CTC	5.32	Sat Fat	5.01
Total Carbs	7.66	Protein	6.89
Fiber	2.34	Calories	195
Total Fat	16.22		

strawberry and toasted almond parfait

For ultimate gratification, very ripe strawberries really matter here. The synergy of these 3 ingredients almost tastes like cake.

24   ounces ripe medium-large strawberries
3   tablespoons slivered almonds
1   cup light whipped topping

Cut the green tops off the strawberries. Slice the strawberries lengthwise, about ⅛" thick.

In a small nonstick skillet over medium heat, cook the almonds about 1 minute, stirring constantly, until golden brown. Let cool.

Fill 4 wine glasses halfway with strawberries. Top each with 2 tablespoons whipped topping. Fill the glasses with the remaining berries and top with the remaining whipped topping. Scatter the almonds on top and serve immediately.

Serves 4

nutritionist's note: Buy a light whipped topping with no unhealthy trans fats. Strawberries are a good source of fiber and antioxidants.

CTC	Total Carbs	Fiber	Total Fat	Sat Fat	Protein	Calories
11.08	14.94	3.86	5.09	2.22	1.95	112

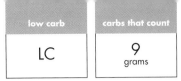
strawberry-cheese brûlée

Is it possible to have a cheesecakelike experience with only 3 ingredients? Well, here it is, and it's surprisingly good for you because I've held the calories down along with the carbs. Whipped cottage cheese is a recently introduced product you'll find in your supermarket's dairy section. You can substitute 1% cottage cheese.

16   ounces ripe small strawberries
6   tablespoons granulated sugar substitute
1⅓   cups whipped cottage cheese

Preheat the broiler.

Cut the green tops off the strawberries. Cut the strawberries in half lengthwise.

Evenly distribute the strawberries among 4 small ovenproof dishes. (Ceramic crème brûlée dishes are perfect for this.) Sprinkle each dish of strawberries with ½ tablespoon of the sugar substitute.

In a food processor, place the whipped cottage cheese. Add 3 tablespoons sugar substitute and begin to process until smooth. Add 2 to 3 tablespoons cold water and continue to process until thick and ultrasmooth. Evenly spread the sweetened cheese over the strawberries and lightly dust with the remaining sugar substitute.

Place the ovenproof dishes on a baking sheet and place under the broiler, about 6" from the heat. Broil until the tops are lightly browned. (Do not overcook because the cheese will begin to "break.") Remove from the oven and let cool to room temperature before serving.

Serves 4

CTC	Total Carbs	Fiber	Total Fat	Sat Fat	Protein	Calories
8.93	11.21	2.28	1.03	.35	11.24	99

melon balls in lime syrup

This is especially refreshing on a hot day. For a great taste thrill, add a pinch of salt and a bit of cracked black pepper (2 "free" ingredients). For a festive presentation, I make several sizes of melon balls and mix them together.

4	cups cantaloupe balls
2	limes
3	tablespoons granulated sugar substitute

In a large bowl, place the cantaloupe balls. Grate the zest of the limes to get 1 tablespoon zest and set aside.

Halve the limes and squeeze to get 3 tablespoons juice. In a small bowl, combine the lime juice with the sugar substitute. Stir until the sugar substitute dissolves. Pour the syrup over the cantaloupe. Add a pinch of salt and toss to combine.

Transfer the cantaloupe and juices to 4 chilled wine glasses. Dust with the lime zest and top with a bit of cracked black pepper. Serve immediately.

Serves 4

nutritionist's note: Cantaloupe contains the antioxidants vitamin C and beta-carotene, what some nutritionists call the "dynamic duo."

CTC	Total Carbs	Fiber	Total Fat	Sat Fat	Protein	Calories
15.58	17.20	1.62	.51	.13	1.63	70

spiced mangoes with coconut

This is a great combination of tastes and color, no matter which spice you choose to use. It also is deliciously different if you don't toast the coconut. Be sure to buy unsweetened shredded coconut. Many supermarket brands are full of added sugar.

⅓	cup unsweetened shredded coconut
4	cups sliced ripe mangoes
1½	teaspoons ground cinnamon or cardamom

In a small nonstick skillet over high heat, toast the coconut, stirring constantly with a wooden spoon or flexible rubber spatula, until golden, about 1 minute. (The coconut will continue to brown briefly after you remove it from the heat, so do not overcook.)

On each of 6 large plates, arrange the mangoes in overlapping slices to cover the interior portion of each plate. Lightly dust the mangoes with cinnamon or cardamom and let sit for 5 minutes. Sprinkle with the toasted coconut and serve.

Serves 6

CTC	Total Carbs	Fiber	Total Fat	Sat Fat	Protein	Calories
18.09	22.06	3.97	7.68	6.62	1.30	152

maple plum compote with mint

You want firm, juicy plums for this recipe, preferably Santa Rosa plums with a purplish-red exterior and yellowish interior. Cook the fruit until it's soft and yielding, but not falling apart. Fat- and sugar-free maple-flavored syrup is one of the few "fake" foods that taste okay, provided it's judiciously combined with delicious fresh ingredients.

8   firm red plums (about 2 pounds)
6   tablespoons sugar-free maple-flavored syrup
1   bunch mint

Halve the plums and remove the pits. Cut each half into 3 wedges. Transfer the plums to a 4-quart saucepan with a cover.

Add 3 tablespoons of the syrup and 3 tablespoons water to the saucepan and bring to a rapid boil. Cook over high heat, stirring constantly, for 5 minutes. Reduce the heat to medium and cover the saucepan. Cook until the plums are quite soft but still retain their shape, 8 to 10 minutes, depending on the firmness of the plums. Let cool in the saucepan.

Cut the mint into fine strips. Transfer the plums, while still slightly warm, and their juices, which will be thick, to shallow bowls. Scatter the mint on top and serve immediately.

Serves 6

nutritionist's note: Check the labels of the sugar-free maple-flavored syrups and buy one sweetened with Splenda, not with sugar alcohols such as sorbitol, maltitol, and manitol. I use one known as Vermont Sugar Free; it's from Maple Grove Farms of Vermont and has 4 carbs per ¼-cup serving.

CTC	Total Carbs	Fiber	Total Fat	Sat Fat	Protein	Calories
15.71	17.95	2.24	.72	.06	1.03	71

honeydew with "sugared" blueberries

This may not be much of a recipe, but it gives you an idea how wonderful "simple" can taste, provided your fruit is ripe.

1   ripe medium honeydew, chilled
1½   cups blueberries
2½   tablespoons granulated sugar substitute

Halve the melon and scoop out the seeds. Cut each melon half into 3 wedges to get 6 wedges. Place 1 melon wedge on each of 6 large dessert plates.

Put the blueberries in a bowl, sprinkle with 2 tablespoons of the sugar substitute, and let sit for 10 minutes.

Divide the blueberries atop the melon wedges. Sprinkle with the remaining ½ tablespoon sugar substitute and serve immediately.

Serves 6

nutritionist's note: Blueberries are considered the "wonder fruit" for their anthocyanins, the natural dyes in food that are revered for their antioxidant powers.

CTC	Total Carbs	Fiber	Total Fat	Sat Fat	Protein	Calories
18.31	20.16	1.85	.29	.05	.98	85

nectarines and blueberries with blueberry syrup

This is a lovely, simple dish for company, and it looks great served in a wine goblet. Fresh peaches can be substituted.

1¾ cups blueberries

3 tablespoons granulated sugar substitute

4 nectarines

In a small saucepan, combine 1 cup of the blueberries, ½ cup water, and 2 tablespoons of the sugar substitute. Bring to a rapid boil. Boil for 2 minutes, then reduce the heat to medium. Cook, stirring constantly, until the sauce gets thick, about 5 minutes. Lightly mash the blueberries to incorporate them into the juices. When the sauce has thickened, remove from the heat and let cool.

Halve the nectarines and carefully remove the pits. Cut the nectarines into thin wedges and place in a bowl. Toss with the remaining ¾ cup blueberries and the remaining 1 tablespoon sugar substitute. Evenly divide the mixture among 4 wine glasses. Drizzle with the blueberry syrup and serve.

Serves 6

CTC	Total Carbs	Fiber	Total Fat	Sat Fat	Protein	Calories
14.57	17.16	2.59	.58	.06	1.14	68

cantaloupe and raspberries with raspberry coulis

You can make this simply by filling melon wedges with raspberries and drizzling the ruby red sauce on top. Or for a restaurant-style presentation that's great for a party, try the alternative preparation detailed below, which will give you little cakelike treats that look like they are studded with gumdrops. The clear, vibrant raspberry sauce is known as a "coulis."

2   pints raspberries
¼   cup granulated sugar substitute
1   large ripe cantaloupe

In a small saucepan, combine 1 pint of the raspberries with the sugar substitute and 1⅓ cups water. Bring to a rapid boil, then reduce the heat and simmer for 20 minutes. Strain through a fine-mesh sieve into a small bowl, pressing down firmly on the raspberries to release all the liquid. Discard the pulp in the sieve. Cover the raspberry sauce and chill until ready to serve.

Halve the melon, remove the seeds, and cut each half into 3 wedges. On each of 6 plates, place a wedge of melon and fill the cavities with the remaining pint of raspberries. Drizzle the sauce on top of the raspberries and around the melon and serve.

Alternatively, you can cut the flesh away from the melon rind and discard the rind. Carefully dice the melon into ¼" cubes. Pack the cubes into ring molds (about 3½" across × 1½" deep; you can make your own molds by removing the top and bottom from very thoroughly washed 6-ounce cans of tuna). Unmold the cubes on large dessert plates, taking care to raise the ring molds slowly so the melon will stay together in a cake shape. Cover the tops of the "cakes" with raspberries, rounded side up. Drizzle the sauce on top and serve.

Serves 6

nutritionist's note: Raspberries are an indulgent way to get fiber and a good dose of antioxidants. They contain only 3 CTC per half cup, so eat as many as you can afford.

CTC	Total Carbs	Fiber	Total Fat	Sat Fat	Protein	Calories
14.84	21.50	6.66	.83	.11	1.94	88

fresh raspberries with lemon-maple sauce

This is a simple and sophisticated merger of flavors that is indeed more than the sum of its parts. Serve it in chilled martini glasses with a lemon twist, and you'll get oohs and ahhs at the table.

3	pints raspberries
½	cup sugar-free maple-flavored syrup
1	lemon

Place the raspberries in a bowl.

In a small bowl, place the syrup. Grate the zest of the lemon and set aside. Halve the lemon and squeeze to get 3 tablespoons juice. Mix the juice into the syrup and stir until combined. Pour the lemon-syrup sauce over the raspberries and let marinate for 15 minutes.

Distribute the raspberries among 4 chilled martini or wine glasses. Top with the sauce from the bowl. Scatter the lemon zest on top and serve immediately. You may also garnish each serving with a long twist of lemon zest or a paper-thin lemon slice cut from an additional lemon.

Serves 4

nutritionist's note: Blueberries lead the list of antioxidant-fortified fruits, but strawberries and raspberries are close to the top.

CTC	Total Carbs	Fiber	Total Fat	Sat Fat	Protein	Calories
11.90	24.81	12.91	1.02	.04	1.77	115

peaches 'n' cream with toasted pecans

This tastes a little like a peach shortcake, without the you-know-what. If the peaches are ripe and juicy, you will hardly miss the cake. Serve it immediately or the whipped topping will dissolve.

½   cup chopped pecans
4   ripe medium peaches
1   cup light whipped topping

In a small nonstick skillet over medium-high heat, cook the pecans, about 1 minute, stirring constantly, until the nuts are toasted and you detect a nutty fragrance. Set aside.

Halve the peaches and remove the pits. Cut each peach into 10 wedges. In each of 4 shallow soup bowls or in dessert cups, place 10 peach wedges. Spray ¼ cup whipped topping on each serving and mix lightly to incorporate. Scatter with the toasted pecans and serve immediately.

Serves 4

CTC	Total Carbs	Fiber	Total Fat	Sat Fat	Protein	Calories
13.55	16.94	3.39	12.79	2.93	2.05	185

peaches in red wine

You can use almost any red wine for this summery dish. Merlot is good, but so is Pinot Noir or Chianti. The funny and fabulous thing is that when you add Splenda to red wine, you get a very good approximation of lambrusco, a sweet, fizzy wine from Italy. Use the most fragrant fruit possible. And yes, you may substitute nectarines for the peaches. White peaches also are lovely.

4   ripe medium peaches
2   cups dry red wine, chilled
¼   cup granulated sugar substitute

Halve the peaches and remove the pits. Cut the peaches into very thin wedges. Evenly distribute the peaches among 4 large wine glasses.

In a large measuring cup, combine the wine and sugar substitute, mixing well. Pour the mixture over the peaches. Serve immediately or cover and refrigerate for up to 30 minutes.

Serves 4

CTC	Total Carbs	Fiber	Total Fat	Sat Fat	Protein	Calories
12.42	14.38	1.96	.09	.01	.92	135

grapefruit with a cherry on top

This may be a bit old-fashioned, but it really is good for you. It's not a bad way to start a meal, either. It is especially pretty when served on unsprayed lemon leaves, which can be purchased at many florists.

2   medium white grapefruits
2   tablespoons granulated sugar substitute
8   fresh cherries, with stems

Halve the grapefruits through their equators. Using a small knife or a grapefruit knife, cut between the membranes to loosen the sections. Sprinkle each grapefruit half with ½ tablespoon (or less) sugar substitute.

Top each grapefruit half with 2 cherries and serve.

Serves 4

CTC	Total Carbs	Fiber	Total Fat	Sat Fat	Protein	Calories
14.27	16.41	2.14	.30	.05	1.21	72

indulgent low carb	carbs that count	low carb	carbs that count
ILC	11.5 grams (strawberries)	LC	10 grams (raspberries)

fresh berries with sweet "crème fraîche"

You may use sweet, ripe strawberries or raspberries for this dessert. Crème fraîche, which is a kind of very rich, fattening sour cream made in France, is made here with yogurt and lightly sweetened. It is so much better than most sweetened yogurts you can buy, for they're filled with artificial flavors and ingredients that surely would embarrass the berries.

3   cups thickly sliced strawberries or whole raspberries
1   cup low-fat plain yogurt
3   tablespoons granulated sugar substitute

If using strawberries, remove the green tops. Reserve a couple of small whole berries for garnish. In 4 shallow dessert bowls, evenly distribute the remaining berries. Lightly sprinkle each serving with ½ teaspoon sugar substitute.

In a bowl, combine the yogurt and remaining 2 tablespoons plus 1 teaspoon sugar substitute, mixing well. (Add a little more sugar substitute to taste, if necessary.) Pour the yogurt over the fruit. Garnish with a strawberry or a raspberry and serve immediately.

Serves 4

nutritionist's note: Some low-carbing folks have been told to stay away from yogurt, opting instead for sour cream because it has fewer carbs. I disagree! While yogurt does have 4 CTC more per serving, the savings of 12 grams saturated fat makes yogurt a far better choice.

strawberries

CTC	Total Carbs	Fiber	Total Fat	Sat Fat	Protein	Calories
11.51	14.37	2.86	1.34	.52	3.76	82

raspberries

CTC	Total Carbs	Fiber	Total Fat	Sat Fat	Protein	Calories
10.03	16.30	6.27	1.38	.52	3.84	90

"stir-fried" strawberries with strawberry sorbet

Here's an unusual way to treat strawberries. They're "stir-fried," not in oil but in a syrup that infuses them with complementary maple-caramel overtones. The resultant juices are delicious. In this recipe, the cooked berries accompany a slushy sorbet for both textural and temperature contrast.

5   pints ripe strawberries
¼   cup sugar-free maple-flavored syrup
½   cup + 2 tablespoons granulated sugar substitute

Up to 1 day before you plan to serve, remove the green tops from 2 pints of the strawberries. In a food processor, process these strawberries with 1 cup water, 1 tablespoon of the syrup, and ½ cup of the sugar substitute until smooth. (You can strain the mixture through a sieve to make the sorbet completely smooth, but I like a bit of texture.) Transfer the mixture to a bowl, chill in the refrigerator for several hours, then freeze in an ice cream machine according to the manufacturer's directions.

When ready to serve, remove the green tops from the remaining 3 pints strawberries. Set aside 6 of the smallest strawberries as a garnish. Cut the remaining berries in half (if small) or in quarters (if large).

In a large nonstick skillet over high heat, heat the remaining 3 tablespoons syrup until hot. Add the strawberries and cook until they are softened but still retain their shape, about 2 minutes. Taste and stir in a bit of sugar substitute, if needed. Remove from the heat and let cool.

Spoon the strawberries and juices into 6 flat-rimmed soup plates or wine glasses. Top each with a scoop of sorbet. Garnish each with a reserved berry.

Serves 6

CTC	Total Carbs	Fiber	Total Fat	Sat Fat	Protein	Calories
13.99	19.51	5.52	.89	.05	1.46	92

mixed berry sherbet

I love the old-fashioned notion of fruit sherbets. This one is an attractive dark raspberry color and is both creamy and dreamy.

⅓	cup granulated sugar substitute
12	ounces frozen unsweetened mixed berries
½	cup light cream

In a blender, dissolve the sugar substitute in ½ cup water. Add the frozen berries and process until smooth. Add the cream and blend well. Freeze the mixture in an ice cream maker according to the manufacturer's directions. Scoop into small wine glasses or small decorative dessert dishes and serve immediately.

Serves 4

nutritionist's note: Once you taste this, you will never go back to the chemical-laden, fat-filled, low-carb frozen ice creams and sorbets on the market today.

CTC	Total Carbs	Fiber	Total Fat	Sat Fat	Protein	Calories
9.57	11.36	1.79	5.89	3.61	1.18	88

lemon-buttermilk sorbet

This sweetly tart, refreshing sorbet is creamy like ice cream and is sure to become your passion. You may substitute fresh lime juice and add bits of cracked black pepper for an exhilarating ending to a rich meal. In that spirit, in very small portions, it also makes a great intermezzo between courses of a formal meal.

4	large lemons
1½	cups granulated sugar substitute
1	quart buttermilk

The day before you plan to serve, grate the zest of 2 or 3 lemons to get 2 tablespoons zest and set aside. Squeeze as many lemons as needed to get ½ cup juice.

In a medium bowl, place the sugar substitute. Add the lemon juice and stir until the sugar substitute is dissolved.

Using a wire whisk, whisk in the buttermilk. Add a pinch of salt and the lemon zest. Whisk until the sugar substitute is completely dissolved and the mixture is smooth. Cover and chill in the refrigerator for several hours or overnight. Freeze the mixture in an ice cream maker according to the manufacturer's directions.

Serves 10

CTC	Total Carbs	Fiber	Total Fat	Sat Fat	Protein	Calories
9.81	9.95	.14	.86	.54	3.27	60

coffee granita with whipped cream

This is a beloved snack in Italy that provides a slushy jolt of caffeine. For the most flavor, make a robust brew from hazelnut-scented or French vanilla coffee beans, or you can use brewed espresso. If you crave the taste of ice-cream parlor whipped topping, you may substitute ½ cup of light whipped topping for the heavy cream.

3   cups hot, double-strength hazelnut or French vanilla brewed coffee or espresso

⅓   cup + 1 tablespoon granulated sugar substitute

7   tablespoons heavy cream

In a pitcher or bowl, place the hot coffee. Add ⅓ cup of the sugar substitute and stir until completely dissolved. Let the mixture cool to room temperature.

Transfer the coffee mixture to a shallow metal baking pan and place in the freezer. Using a large fork, stir the mixture every 30 minutes to break up the ice crystals. Continue to do this for about 3 hours, until the mixture is frozen and the ice crystals are uniform.

When ready to serve, in a bowl with a wire whisk, whip the cream and the remaining 1 tablespoon sugar substitute, until the mixture is thick and stands in soft peaks. Spoon the granita into 4 chilled wine glasses and top with the whipped cream. Sprinkle with a little ground coffee, if desired.

Serves 4

CTC	Total Carbs	Fiber	Total Fat	Sat Fat	Protein	Calories
4.65	4.65	0	9.65	6.01	.71	108

frozen hot chocolate

This slushy drink qua *dessert was derived from one made famous at New York's Serendipity restaurant. You need to serve it with both a spoon and a straw.*

½   cup unsweetened Dutch process cocoa
¾   cup granulated sugar substitute
2½   cups 1% milk

Up to 1 day before you plan to serve, into a medium saucepan and using a small strainer, sift the cocoa to remove any lumps. Add the sugar substitute and ½ cup of the milk and stir to form a smooth paste. Using a whisk, slowly add the remaining 2 cups milk and cook over medium heat, whisking constantly, until the ingredients are thoroughly incorporated and the mixture is smooth, 2 to 3 minutes. Let cool off the heat, then pour the mixture into an ice cube tray and freeze for a minimum of 8 hours.

Before serving, put the blender canister in the freezer to chill for 1 hour. Remove the frozen cubes and add to the chilled blender canister. Add 2 tablespoons water and, beginning on low speed, break up the cubes, then increase to high speed and process until smooth and slushy. (This will take several minutes.) Serve immediately in frozen coffee cups or chilled wine glasses.

Serves 4

CTC	Total Carbs	Fiber	Total Fat	Sat Fat	Protein	Calories
14.06	17.63	3.57	3.09	1.87	7.12	106

italian zabaglione

This classic Italian dessert from northern Italy lends itself almost effortlessly to a low-carb regime. The secret is to whip as much air as possible into the warm egg yolks so they expand into a billowy cloud.

5	extra-large egg yolks
¼	cup granulated sugar substitute
⅓	cup dry Marsala

Fill a 4-quart pot one-third of the way with water. Bring the water to a boil, then immediately reduce the heat to a simmer. Choose a large metal bowl that will fit above the pot comfortably. With the bowl still on the counter, add the egg yolks, sugar substitute, and Marsala. Using a wire balloon whisk, whisk the ingredients together until incorporated.

Place the bowl on the pot of simmering water. Whisk constantly until the mixture becomes very light and begins to thicken. Make sure the water below remains at a simmer. Continue to whisk, incorporating as much air as possible, until the egg mixture begins to look like whipped heavy cream and comes away from the sides of the bowl, about 5 minutes total. (Be careful not to overbeat or overheat, because the mixture can turn into scrambled eggs very quickly. You can also do this with a hand-held electric mixer, but I find I can incorporate more air using a big whisk.)

Spoon the warm thickened mixture into 4 small wine glasses and serve immediately.

Serves 4

CTC	Total Carbs	Fiber	Total Fat	Sat Fat	Protein	Calories
2.28	2.28	0	7.69	2.38	4.21	109

sweet orange roulade

My dear friend, Sally-Jo O'Brien, who often tests my recipes, loved this recipe (even with the sugar substitute) and prepares it as a treat for her young daughter, Julia. It's sweet, citrusy, and custardlike and is great for Sunday brunch.

4	large oranges
5	extra-large eggs
½	cup granulated sugar substitute

Preheat the oven to 450°F.

Thoroughly coat an 8" × 8" glass baking dish with cooking spray.

Grate the zest of enough oranges to get 2 heaping tablespoons. Halve 2 of the oranges and squeeze to get ½ cup juice. With a sharp knife, cut the rind from the remaining oranges. Discard the rind. Slice the oranges crosswise into thin rounds or cut between the membranes to release the segments. Set aside.

In a medium bowl, combine the eggs, sugar substitute, orange juice, zest, and a pinch of salt. With an electric mixer on high speed, beat for 1 minute. Pour the mixture into the prepared baking dish and bake for 15 minutes, until the top is puffed and golden brown. Remove from the oven and let cool for 5 minutes.

Meanwhile, place a clean linen kitchen towel on a board large enough to accommodate the baked custard. Lightly dampen the towel with water. Using a small, sharp knife, cut the custard around the edges to loosen. Place the board on top of the pan, towel side down, then turn everything over together and invert the custard onto the towel. Remove the pan. Lift half of the towel and use it to roll up the firm custard, jelly roll–style, about 1½ times. Press down lightly. Gently lift the roulade from the towel and place on a large plate.

Garnish with the reserved oranges. Serve slightly warm, at room temperature, or cold.

Serves 4

CTC	Total Carbs	Fiber	Total Fat	Sat Fat	Protein	Calories
15.76	18.30	2.54	6.38	1.95	8.84	164

peanut thins

Crisp and nicely balanced with sweet and peanutty tastes, these will definitely satisfy any cookie craving you might have. Make sure you use natural peanut butter since nonnatural brands contain sugar and hydrogenated vegetable oils.

1   cup granulated sugar substitute
1   extra-large egg
1   cup natural super-chunky peanut butter

In a bowl, combine the sugar substitute and 2 tablespoons cold water. With an electric mixer, mix until smooth. Add the egg and a pinch of salt and mix well.

Pour off most of the separated oil, if any, from the jar of peanut butter and stir the remaining contents of the jar well. Add 1 cup peanut butter to the egg mixture and blend thoroughly. Wrap tightly in plastic wrap and refrigerate for 1 hour.

Meanwhile, preheat the oven to 375°F.

Line a baking sheet with parchment paper.

Scoop out 2 teaspoons dough at a time and roll into balls about 1" in diameter. Place on the lined baking sheet and, using the tines of a fork, flatten the balls into disks about 1¼" in diameter.

Bake for 10 to 11 minutes, or until just firm to the touch. (Do not bake too long or the cookies will burn.) Remove from the oven and let the cookies cool on the baking sheet. Store in a tightly covered tin up to 2 days.

Makes 24 cookies (data is per cookie)

nutritionist's note: These are higher in protein and have far fewer carbs than the average store-bought cookie.

CTC	Total Carbs	Fiber	Total Fat	Sat Fat	Protein	Calories
2.69	3.36	.67	5.54	1.06	2.59	70

maple-walnut tea cakes

I love these little tea cakes and so does my husband, who generally does not care for such things. He enjoys them with his morning coffee and his afternoon cup of tea. Either way, it's a great low-carb treat (even if you have 2!) and a cinch to make.

8   ounces walnuts halves (about 2 cups)

2   extra-large eggs, room temperature

½   cup sugar-free maple-flavored syrup

Preheat the oven to 375°F.

Line a 12-muffin tin with fluted muffin papers.

In a large nonstick skillet over medium-low heat, cook the walnuts, stirring constantly, until the nuts are lightly toasted and smell nutty, about 4 minutes. Remove from the heat. When completely cooled, place in a food processor and process until finely ground. Set aside.

Pour boiling water into the bowl of an electric mixer to warm it (which helps to increase the volume of the eggs when beaten). Pour out the water and thoroughly dry the bowl. Break the eggs into the warm bowl and add the syrup and a pinch of salt. With an electric mixer, beat on high speed until the mixture is very thick and has increased in volume, 6 to 7 minutes.

Using a flexible rubber spatula, fold the ground walnuts into the beaten eggs. Evenly distribute the mixture among the 12 muffin cups.

Bake for about 35 minutes, or until the cakes are just set. (Use a wooden skewer to test for doneness; the skewer should be dry when removed from the cake.) Remove from the oven and let cool. These can be stored in a tightly covered tin for up to 2 days.

Makes 12 (data is per cake)

nutritionist's note: Walnuts are low in saturated fat and an excellent source of omega-3 and omega-6 fatty acids. Research has found that eating regular amounts of walnuts (and almonds, too) reduces the bad cholesterol (LDL) in the blood.

CTC	Total Carbs	Fiber	Total Fat	Sat Fat	Protein	Calories
2.12	3.39	1.27	13.16	1.42	3.92	149

chocolate-tahini cups

These superb little candies will become your signature offering after dinner. You need to buy little 1" paper liners, generally used for candy (they look like tiny muffin liners), at any specialty baking or party store. Use a great dark chocolate, such as Scharffen Berger, from California, which is available in many specialty food shops and good supermarkets.

¼ cup tahini (sesame seed paste)
¼ cup granulated sugar substitute
8 ounces good-quality 70% bittersweet chocolate

Stir the tahini and its oil together in the jar, in case it has separated. In a medium bowl, place the tahini and stir until smooth.

In a small bowl, stir the sugar substitute in 2 teaspoons water until dissolved. Stir this mixture into the tahini and mix thoroughly.

Coarsely chop the chocolate and put in the top of a double boiler. Set the top over simmering water, making sure the bottom of the double boiler doesn't touch the water. Pour all but 1 tablespoon of the sweetened tahini into the top of the double boiler with the chocolate. Stir until the chocolate is melted and the tahini has been thoroughly incorporated. Remove from the heat.

Spoon the chocolate mixture into twenty-four 1" fluted paper candy cups. Let cool for 5 minutes. To decorate the candies, dip the tip of a toothpick into the remaining tablespoon of sweetened tahini and swirl it into the tops of the candies. Refrigerate until set. Store, covered and refrigerated, for up to 1 week.

Makes 24 (data is per candy)

nutritionist's note: Most low-carb chocolates on the market are filled with sugar alcohols that can wreak havoc on your stomach. These chocolate cups have nothing but great taste.

CTC	Total Carbs	Fiber	Total Fat	Sat Fat	Protein	Calories
6.57	6.88	.31	7.27	3.69	1.54	99

chocolate-dipped strawberries

This is the ultimate reward for good behavior. It feels indulgent, yet, improbably enough, it fits into our low-carb category. Toasting the coconut deepens the flavor, but if you're in a hurry, you can skip the toasting step.

16   very large strawberries, with their stems (about 1 pound)
3   tablespoons unsweetened shredded coconut
3½   ounces good-quality 70% bittersweet chocolate

Wash the berries and carefully pat dry with paper towels. (Moisture on the strawberries will cause the chocolate to clump up, so do not rush the drying.) Leave the stems on for easy dipping.

In a small nonstick skillet over medium heat, toast the coconut, stirring constantly, until the coconut just begins to turn golden brown, 1 to 2 minutes. Immediately transfer the coconut to a small bowl and let cool.

Break the chocolate into pieces and put in the top of a double boiler over simmering water. Stirring occasionally, carefully heat the chocolate until it just melts into a smooth sauce.

Line a large plate with waxed paper. Remove the top of the double boiler. Dip each strawberry about three-quarters of the way up the berry into the chocolate. Immediately put each dipped strawberry on the lined plate. Lightly sprinkle with toasted coconut. Let cool until the chocolate completely hardens, then serve.

Makes 16 (data is per strawberry)

nutritionist's note: Bittersweet chocolate is now known to be a prime source of antioxidants, which subdue harmful free radicals in our bodies.

CTC	Total Carbs	Fiber	Total Fat	Sat Fat	Protein	Calories
4.28	5.33	1.05	4.61	3.23	.81	64

snacks and menus

50 super snacks

Many low-carbers find that snacking is one of their biggest challenges. Packaged products abound, but protein bars, for example, are typically overly processed and full of chemicals and sugar alcohols, while a chunk of processed lunch meat like bologna may have no carbs, but it's loaded with saturated fat. Here we offer real choices, real food: 50 low-carb super snacks. All fit into one of our three categories, ranging from 0 to 18 grams CTC (VLC—very low carb, LC—low carb, or ILC—indulgent low carb). Better yet, each complete snack has fewer than 250 calories—less than a container of low-fat yogurt with fruit or a 2-ounce bag of chips.

You should also look at the Party Food chapter (page 41) for additional low-carb options: a handful of Glazed Walnuts (page 50), some Smoked Salmon Pâté with Pita Crisps (page 54), or a plate of Rosemary Meatballs (page 63)—all make for great snacking during the day.

Note that each snack recipe below yields 1 serving, except where noted.

very low carb (0 to 5 grams ctc)

#1
CTC = 4 grams Calories = 222

1 soft-boiled egg
2 slices crisp bacon
½ cup 1% low-fat cottage cheese

Put the egg in an egg cup and place it on a small plate with the bacon and cottage cheese.

#2
CTC = 4 grams Calories = 98

½ red bell pepper
3 radishes
1 ounce feta cheese

Cut the pepper into ¼-inch-wide strips. Trim the radishes and cut in half lengthwise. Arrange on small plate with the cheese.

#3
CTC = 4 grams Calories = 144

3 ounces sliced turkey breast or Black Forest ham
3 medium leaves butter lettuce
2 small jarred pickled peppers

Roll the turkey or ham in lettuce leaves to make 3 packets. Place on a small plate with the peppers alongside.

#4

CTC = 2 grams Calories = 190

3 ounces flank steak, grilled and thinly sliced
1 ounce mache or arugula
2 teaspoons balsamic vinegar

Arrange the slices of steak, either warm or cold, in overlapping pattern on a small plate. Top with a mound of mache or arugula that has been washed and dried well. Splash with the vinegar.

#5

CTC = 2 grams Calories = 193

1 kirby cucumber
½ tablespoon lemon-flavored olive oil
3 ounces store-bought gravlax or smoked salmon, thinly sliced

Peel the cucumber and slice paper thin. Toss with the oil, salt, and pepper, and mound in the center of a small plate. Arrange the salmon slices on top.

#6

CTC = .5 gram Calories = 159

1 ounce watercress, stems trimmed
3 ounces poached salmon, chilled
1 lemon wedge

Scatter the watercress in the center of a small plate. Place the salmon on top and serve with the lemon wedge.

#7

CTC = 5 grams Calories = 195

½ ripe medium peach, thinly sliced
1 ounce fresh goat cheese (chèvre)
½ ounce pecan halves, lightly toasted

Fan out the peach slices on a small plate. Arrange the goat cheese next to the peaches and scatter the pecans over the fruit and cheese.

#8

CTC = 2 grams Calories = 95

2 thin slices low-fat Muenster cheese
2 large butter lettuce leaves
2 dill pickle spears

Lay each cheese slice on a lettuce leaf, place a pickle spear in the center, and roll up to get 2 wraps.

#9

CTC = 1.5 grams Calories = 131

2 hard-boiled eggs
2 tablespoons light mayonnaise
2 teaspoons mustard

Boil the eggs and chill. Peel the eggs and cut them in half lengthwise. Remove the yolks and mash with the mayonnaise, mustard, salt, and freshly ground black pepper. Fill the whites with the yolk mixture.

Serves 2

#10

CTC = 2 grams Calories = 180

1 large stalk celery
1 ounce blue cheese
2 tablespoons Neufchâtel cheese

Cut the celery into 3" lengths. Finely chop the leaves. In a bowl, mash the cheeses together. Using a small spoon or knife, stuff the celery with the cheese. Sprinkle with the chopped celery leaves.

#11

CTC = 2.5 grams Calories = 96

½ small tomato, sliced
4 small black olives
1 ounce feta cheese, crumbled

Arrange the tomato slices and olives on a small plate and scatter the cheese over top.

#12

CTC = 2.5 grams Calories = 121

1 cup cooked broccoli florets
1 ounce shredded low-fat cheddar cheese
Sprinkling curry powder

Preheat the broiler. Put the broccoli in a small ovenproof dish. Sprinkle with salt and freshly ground black pepper. Top with the cheese and curry powder. Broil until bubbly.

#13

CTC = 5 grams Calories = 70

2 tablespoons prepared hummus
½ cup sliced jícama
1 wedge lime

Put the hummus in the center of a small plate. Surround with the jícama slices for dipping. Season with cracked pepper and serve with the lime.

#14

CTC = 4.5 grams Calories = 173

1½ tablespoons light mayonnaise
2 teaspoons prepared white horseradish
3 ounces boiled shrimp, chilled

In a bowl, mix the mayonnaise with the horseradish. Serve with the shrimp.

#15

CTC = 1.5 grams Calories = 232

6 extra-large eggs
3 tablespoons light mayonnaise
1 can (7 ounces) white tuna in oil, drained

Boil the eggs. Chill. Peel the eggs and mash with the mayonnaise and tuna. Add salt and pepper to taste. Chill.

Serves 4

#16

CTC = 4.5 grams Calories = 238

1 glass (5 ounces) dry sparkling wine
3 medium strawberries
¾ ounce almonds

Pour the sparkling wine into a chilled champagne glass. Serve with the strawberries and almonds.

#17

CTC = 4 grams Calories = 245

1 glass (5 ounces) dry red wine
3 ounces rare roast beef
1 tablespoon Dijon mustard

Serve a glass of red wine with a plate of roast beef mounded high, sprinkled with coarse salt and with a dab of mustard on the side.

#18

CTC = 4 grams Calories = 190

1 glass (5 ounces) dry rosé wine
½ small red pepper
1 ounce soft goat cheese with herbs

Chill the wine and pour into a glass. Cut the pepper into ½-inch-thick wedges. Mound a bit of cheese on each wedge.

#19

CTC = 5 grams Calories = 191

1 can (6 ounces) albacore tuna in water
1 tablespoon white balsamic vinegar
1 tablespoon julienned fresh basil

Drain the tuna and put on a small plate. Sprinkle with the vinegar and top with the basil.

#20

CTC = 3 grams Calories = 176

2 ounces bresaola (air-dried beef)
¼ ripe avocado, thinly sliced
1 wedge lemon

Arrange the bresaola on a small plate. Top with the avocado. Dust with coarsely ground black pepper and serve with the lemon.

#21

CTC = 3 grams Calories = 188

2 ounces grilled Canadian bacon
1 hot, poached egg
¼ cup salsa, warmed

Put the Canadian bacon on a small plate. Top with the poached egg and spoon the salsa on top.

#22

CTC = 4 grams Calories = 163

4 ounces store-bought sashimi
3 tablespoons soy sauce
½ tablespoon wasabi paste

Put the sashimi on a small plate. Put soy sauce in small ramekin and put a mound of wasabi in the center of the soy sauce. Serve with chopsticks.

#23

CTC = 3.5 grams Calories = 229

1 can (3 ounces) salmon
2 tablespoons light
** mayonnaise**
1 teaspoon wasabi paste

In a bowl, mash the salmon with the mayonnaise and wasabi. Chill.

#24

CTC = 3 grams Calories = 171

4 ounces regular tofu
2 teaspoons roasted sesame
** oil**
2 teaspoons soy sauce

Cut the tofu into cubes or slices and place them on a plate. Drizzle with the oil and soy sauce and sprinkle with freshly ground pepper. Alternatively, you can stir-fry the slices of tofu in the sesame oil and sprinkle with soy sauce.

#25

CTC = 4.5 grams Calories = 247

¼ cup low-fat plain yogurt
2 tablespoons finely chopped
** cilantro + cilantro leaves**
4 ounces poached salmon

In a bowl, combine the yogurt and the finely chopped cilantro to make a sauce. Spoon over the salmon. Dust with salt and coarsely black pepper and garnish with the cilantro leaves.

More snacks: You may also choose any recipe in the book that is VLC and under 250 calories.

low carb (6 to 10 grams ctc)

#26

CTC = 8 grams Calories = 200

3 ounces honeydew
1 ounce prosciutto
1 ounce thinly shaved
** Parmesan cheese**

Cut the melon into thin slices and arrange on a plate. Drape the prosciutto over the melon and scatter the cheese on top. Dust with coarsely ground black pepper.

#27

CTC = 8 grams Calories = 116

2 pieces store-bought gefilte
** fish, chilled**
½ ounce mesclun greens
2 tablespoons prepared white
** horseradish**

Put the fish on a small plate. Tuck the greens alongside the fish. Serve with the horseradish.

#28

CTC = 8.5 grams Calories = 228

2 tablespoons freshly ground
** peanut butter**
1 medium stalk celery, cut into
** sticks**
1 small carrot, cut into sticks

Mound the peanut butter in the center of a small plate and surround with the celery and carrots for dipping.

More snacks: You may also choose any recipe in the book that is LC and under 250 calories, which includes several desserts.

#29

CTC = 7 grams Calories = 196

1½ ounces red grapes (about 8 grapes), on their stems
¾ ounce Roquefort cheese
½ ounce walnuts (about 7 halves)

Arrange all of the ingredients on a small plate.

#30

CTC = 7 grams Calories = 189

6 cherries, on their stems
¾ ounce ripe brie
½ ounce hazelnuts, lightly toasted

Arrange all of the ingredients on a small plate.

#31

CTC = 8 grams Calories = 182

½ small apple
1 ounce low-fat sharp cheddar cheese
5 small macadamia nuts (½ ounce)

Slice the apple thinly. Fan out on a small plate. Serve the cheese and nuts alongside.

#32

CTC = 10 grams Calories = 198

½ small ripe pear
1 ounce Parmigiano-Reggiano cheese
4 whole almonds, with skins

Cut the pear into 2 wedges. Cut the cheese into 2 chunks. Place the pear and cheese on a small plate with the nuts.

#33

CTC = 9.5 grams Calories = 136

½ small apple
1 tablespoon natural peanut butter
1 large strawberry, sliced

Cut the apple into 2 thick slices. Spread the apple with the peanut butter and top with strawberry slices.

#34

CTC = 8 grams Calories = 192

½ ripe avocado, skin on
⅓ cup spicy salsa
1 wedge lime

Remove the pit from the avocado. Cut a tiny slice from the rounded bottom of the avocado half so that it sits on a small plate without wobbling. Pour the salsa into the avocado cavity. Serve with the lime.

#35

CTC = 8 grams Calories = 176

½ fennel bulb, thinly sliced
1 tablespoon white balsamic vinegar
1 ounce Asiago cheese

Remove the fronds from the fennel and chop them finely. Arrange the fennel on a small plate. Splash with the vinegar. Slice the cheese paper-thin and scatter over the fennel. Top with the chopped fronds.

#36

CTC = 10 grams Calories = 91

¼ small cantaloupe
⅓ cup 1% low-fat cottage cheese
Fresh mint

Remove the seeds from the cantaloupe. Cut a tiny slice from the rounded bottom of the melon wedge so that it sits on a small plate without wobbling. Fill the cavity with the cottage cheese. Cut the mint into thin strips and scatter on top or simply garnish with a sprig.

#37

CTC = 7.5 grams Calories = 178

½ cup part-skim ricotta cheese
¼ teaspoon vanilla, lemon, or almond extract
2 teaspoons granulated sugar substitute

In a bowl, mix together the cheese, extract, and sugar substitute and chill. Serve in a pretty dessert dish.

indulgent low carb (11 to 18 grams ctc)

#38

CTC = 12 grams Calories = 230

2 poached eggs, hot
1 slice whole wheat toast
½ teaspoon butter

Place the eggs on lightly buttered toast and serve immediately with coarse salt and pepper.

#39

CTC = 11 grams Calories = 239

½ small whole wheat bagel, toasted
2 tablespoons Neufchâtel cheese
3 ounces smoked salmon

Spread the bagel with the Neufchâtel cheese and arrange the salmon on top.

#40

CTC = 12.5 grams Calories = 200

2 small fresh ripe figs
1 ounce Gorgonzola cheese
1 tablespoon pine nuts, lightly toasted

Cut the figs in half through the stem ends. Top each half with a thin slice of cheese. Press the pine nuts on top.

#41

CTC = 15 grams Calories = 137

2 cups canned chickpeas
2 tablespoons garlic olive oil
1 tablespoon dried rosemary leaves, chopped

Drain the chickpeas and pat dry with paper towels. Heat the oil in a large nonstick skillet. Add the chickpeas and rosemary. Cook over high heat for several minutes until crispy. Add salt and freshly ground black pepper to taste.

Serves 6

#42

CTC = 14 grams Calories = 245

⅔ cup low-fat plain yogurt
1 tablespoon extra-virgin olive oil
1 tablespoon za'atar (see page 139)

Put the yogurt in a small bowl. Drizzle with the oil and sprinkle with the za'atar.

#43

CTC = 12 grams Calories = 200

½ whole wheat pita (6" in diameter)
2 ounces thinly sliced turkey breast
1 ounce low-fat shredded cheddar cheese

Preheat the broiler. Split pita into whole rounds. Cover with the turkey and sprinkle evenly with the cheese. Place under the broiler until the cheese is melted and bubbly.

#44

CTC = 14 grams Calories = 144

½ cup low-fat plain yogurt
¼ cup blueberries
1 tablespoon chopped walnuts

Put the yogurt in a small bowl. Add the blueberries and mix until blended. Transfer to a small chilled wine glass and top with the walnuts.

More snacks: Any recipe in this book that is ILC and under 250 calories also makes a good ILC snack. This includes most of the desserts.

#45

CTC = 11 grams Calories = 186

1 cup raspberries
¼ cup light whipped topping
½ ounce toasted sliced
**   almonds**

Put the washed and dried raspberries in a pretty dessert dish. Top with the whipped topping and almonds.

#46

CTC = 11.5 grams Calories = 150

1 cup chicken broth
¼ cup cooked brown rice
¼ cup cooked, cubed chicken
**   breast**

In a small saucepan, heat the broth. Add the rice and chicken and simmer until hot.

#47

CTC = 17 grams Calories = 218

½ cup spicy salsa
½ cup canned black beans
¼ cup shredded low-fat
**   cheddar cheese**

Preheat the oven to 350°F. In a bowl, mix the salsa and drained beans and put in medium ramekin or onion soup bowl. Top with the cheese and bake for 15 minutes, until hot and bubbly.

#48

CTC = 12 grams Calories = 238

1 slice whole wheat bread
1 tablespoon Dijon mustard
1½ ounces hard salami

Toast the bread. Spread with the mustard. Top with the salami.

#49

CTC = 18 grams Calories = 123

1 cup strawberries
2 tablespoons sugar-free
**   maple-flavored syrup**
½ cup low-fat plain yogurt

Quarter the strawberries and toss with 1 tablespoon of the syrup. Put in a wine glass. Top with the yogurt and drizzle with the remaining syrup.

#50

CTC = 11 grams Calories = 191

1 ounce dark chocolate
8 almonds
Freshly brewed espresso, in a
**   demitasse cup**

Nibble chocolate and almonds between sips of espresso.

52 magical menus

The 225 recipes in this book offer an almost limitless number of menu combinations. This section presents 52 that we've compiled for you—for breakfast, lunch, dinner, and holidays. All of the menus are based on an 1,800 calorie day (breakfasts 225 to 369 calories, lunches 268 to 684 calories, dinners 518 to 771 calories, and holiday menus 396 to 836 calories). Every menu fits into one of our three categories (VLC, LC, and ILC), except several of the holiday menus, which still come in under 25 grams of Carbs That Count (CTC).

Even if you chose our highest-calorie menus and had three of them in a day (breakfast, lunch, and a holiday dinner), you would still come in under 1,900 calories—barely breaking your diet! And if you opted for the highest-carb menus, you would consume 53 CTC that day—which is below "maintenance" for many low-carbers and allows you the pleasure of stretching the rules without consequences or guilt.

Our goal is to help you combine our recipes to meet your needs for taste, variety, carbs, and calories. We give you the tools to pick and choose what is right for you and encourage you to make your own "menu magic." One day, you might want to eat a light breakfast because you are having guests for dinner, or you may need to balance a big holiday breakfast with a lower-carb lunch and dinner. Depending on what you choose (all you need to do is add up the CTCs and calories that can be found with each recipe), you could fit in several snacks as well. It's always up to you, and it's always delicious. This simple method will give you the variety you need to make this healthier approach to low-carb eating a way of life, not a passing fad.

What's more, because the following menus are composed entirely of 3-ingredient recipes, you'll always qualify for the express lane at the supermarket!

Most of the menus are based on three courses, but you may augment or change them by adding an hors d'oeuvres, side dish, or dessert of your choosing. Just add up the CTCs, calories, and saturated fat to fit your specifications.

Here are a few general guidelines.

■ You can add a glass of wine to any of the menus:

Dry white or sparkling wine: a 5-ounce glass will add 1 CTC and 100 calories.

Dry red wine: a 5-ounce glass will add 2.5 CTC and 105 calories.

Dry rose wine: a 5-ounce glass will add 2 CTC and 105 calories.

■ You can add any recipe from any of the chapters—Party Food, Soups and Starters, Vegetables and Side Dishes, etc.—to augment any menu. Just add on the number of calories, CTCs, and saturated fat.

■ For dessert, you can add 1 cup of fresh raspberries or fresh halved strawberries. Add sugar substitute to taste and garnish with fresh mint. One cup of raspberries will add 6 grams CTC and 60 calories. One cup of strawberries will add 7 grams CTC and 43 calories. You can add warm Italian Zabaglione (page 254) on top of the berries and only add 2.5 grams CTC and 109 calories. Or add any of the desserts on pages 235 to 259.

■ You can finish any meal with unsweetened coffee or tea. We recommend drinking seltzer or mineral water, or iced tea you make yourself—green, black, or herbal, during the meal. We do not recommend sweetened carbonated beverages.

breakfast menus

very low carb (0 to 5 grams CTC)	Vermont Cheddar Frittata with Pickled Jalapeños (page 22) Homemade Turkey Sausage (page 38) Coffee CTC = 3 grams Calories = 229	Ham 'n' Eggs with Red-Eye Gravy (page 24) garnished with ¼ small orange and 1 small strawberry Iced mint tea with 2 teaspoons sugar substitute CTC = 4.5 grams Calories = 234	Chinese Marbled Eggs (page 27) Five-Spice Bacon (page 37) 1 very thin slice cantaloupe Green tea CTC = 5 grams Calories = 261
low carb (6 to 10 grams CTC)	Frittata with Pancetta and Basil (page 23) Broiled plum tomato 1 Whole Wheat Pita Chip (page 51) Coffee CTC = 6.5 grams Calories = 310	Grapefruit with Cinnamon "Sugar" (page 36) Smoked Fish Plate with lemon cream cheese (page 89) Coffee CTC = 9.5 grams Calories = 225	Fried Eggs, Italian-Style (page 30) 2 ounces thinly sliced bresaola 2 Whole Wheat Pita Chips (page 51) Espresso CTC = 6.5 grams Calories = 357
indulgent low carb (11 to 18 grams CTC)	Poached eggs on buttered toast (2 poached eggs, 1 slice whole wheat bread, and 1 teaspoon butter) Prosciutto-Honeydew-Mint Brochettes (page 57) Tea with lemon CTC = 17 grams Calories = 290	Sweet Orange Roulade (page 255) Five-Spice Bacon (page 37) Coffee CTC = 17 grams Calories = 261	Eggs à la Salsa (page 21) Homemade Turkey Sausage (page 38) ½ whole wheat tortilla Iced mint tea CTC = 17 grams Calories = 369

Stir-Fried Eggs with
    Shiitake Mushrooms
    (page 35)
Homemade Turkey
    Sausage (page 38)
½ small orange
Oolong tea

CTC = 8.5 grams Calories = 311

Poached Egg, Smoked
    Salmon, and Chives
    (page 26)
Strawberry-Cheese Brûleé
    (page 237)
French-press coffee

CTC = 9 grams Calories = 294

Fresh Raspberries with
    Lemon-Maple Sauce
    (page 244)
Eggs and Canadian
    Bacon, My Way
    (page 33)
Espresso

CTC = 13.5 grams Calories = 350

lunch menus

Seared Salmon on Lemony
  Cucumbers (page 97)
Baby Spinach Salad with
  Crispy Bacon
  (page 101)
Iced coffee

CTC = 3.5 grams Calories = 403

Mesclun with Lemon-
  Raspberry Vinaigrette
  (page 95)
Artic Char with Dill and
  Vermouth (page 178)
Steamed Broccoli with
  Stir-Fried Pecans
  (page 193)
French-press coffee

CTC = 5 grams Calories = 531

Chilled Avocado Soup
  (page 69)
Bay-Steamed Halibut with
  Lemon Oil (page 171)
Sautéed Escarole with
  Garlic (page 201)
Coffee

CTC = 4.5 grams Calories = 574

Baby Spinach Salad with
  Crispy Bacon
  (page 101)
Chicken Rollatini with
  Salami and Roasted
  Peppers (page 142)
Simple Fried Cauliflower
  (page 199)
Espresso

CTC = 8 grams Calories = 636

Jade Zucchini Soup with
  Crab (page 76)
Peppered Tuna "Tataki"
  (page 88)
Stir-Fried Spinach with
  Sesame Seeds
  (page 213)
Iced green tea

CTC = 7 grams Calories = 446

Carpaccio of Beef with
  Mustard Mayonnaise
  (page 91)
Basil Shrimp and Crispy
  Pancetta (page 162)
Oven-Roasted Asparagus
  with Fried Capers
  (page 191)
Cannarino (hot water with
  lots of lemon peel)

CTC = 8 grams Calories = 665

Ginger and Chicken
  Consommé (page 72)
Wasabi Salmon
  (page 179)
Sugar Snaps with Yellow
  Pepper Julienne
  (page 215)
Iced green tea

CTC = 13 grams Calories = 571

Chilled Asparagus with
  Creamy Sesame
  Dressing (page 93)
Broiled Veal Steak with
  Fresh Thyme Mustard
  (page 129)
Confit of Carrots and
  Lemon (page 197)
Coffee

CTC = 13 grams Calories = 508

Bibb Lettuce and Roasted
  Pepper Salad with
  Creamy Feta Dressing
  (page 96)
Chardonnay Mussels
  (page 98)
Coffee

CTC = 14 grams Calories = 268

Garlic Soup with Chicken
and Cilantro (page 75)
Prosciutto-Wrapped
Halibut (page 170)
Braised Endive with Bay
Leaves (page 200)
Coffee

CTC = 2 grams Calories = 684

Broccoli Soup with Basil
Butter (page 77)
Warm Poached Chicken
with Sun-Dried Tomatoes
and Capers (page 150)
Asiago-Roasted Fennel
(page 202)
Coffee

CTC = 10 grams Calories = 580

Cream of Cauliflower
soup, chilled (page 81)
Cold Poached Chicken
with Avocado and
Mango (page 152)
Darjeeling tea with lemon

CTC = 17 grams Calories = 432

dinner menus

Wine recommendations are made with each menu but are not included in the analyses. To count a glass or two of wine, see page 42.

very low carb (0 to 5 grams CTC)

Chilled Avocado Soup
(page 69)
Sautéed Striped Bass with
Basil Sauce (page 175)
Simple Fried Cauliflower
(page 199)

CTC = 5.5 grams   Calories = 624

Wine: Chardonnay

Mesclun with Lemon-
Raspberry Vinaigrette
(page 95)
Poulet aux Champignons
(page 135)
Stir-Fried Spinach with
Sesame Seeds
(page 213)

CTC = 5 grams   Calories = 670

Wine: Pinot Noir

Smoked Fish Plate with
Lemon Cream Cheese
(page 89)
Bay Leaf-and-Beef
Brochettes (page 127)
Green Beans with Pesto
and Walnuts (page 204)

CTC = 4.5 grams   Calories = 627

Wine: Chardonnay (from
Australia)

low carb (6 to 10 grams CTC)

Miso Soup with Chorizo
(page 74)
Five-Spice Roasted
Chicken (page 134)
Stir-Fried Spinach with
Sesame Seeds
(page 213)
Shiitake Mushrooms in
Sherry-Pepper Cream
(page 207)

CTC = 10.5 grams   Calories = 622

Wine: Pinot Noir

Jade Zucchini Soup with
Crab (page 76)
Pan-Seared Rib-Eye with
Arugula (page 122)
Almond-Crusted Baked
Tomatoes (page 216)

CTC = 10 grams   Calories = 518

Wine: Chardonnay or
Merlot

Avocado and Crab
"Martini" (page 87)
Broiled Veal Steak with
Fresh Thyme Mustard
(page 129)
Asiago-Roasted Fennel
(page 202)

CTC = 9.5 grams   Calories = 657

Wine: Chardonnay

indulgent low carb (11 to 18 grams CTC)

Broccoli Soup with Basil
Butter (page 77)
Sun-Dried Tomato Meat
Loaf (page 117)
Frenched Beans with
Warm Vinaigrette
(page 203)
Roasted Portabellos on
Rosemary Branches
(page 206)

CTC = 17 grams   Calories = 734

Wine: Merlot

Chilled Asparagus with
Creamy Sesame
Dressing (page 93)
Garlic-Miso Pork Chops
(page 108)
Sugar Snaps with Yellow
Pepper Julienne
(page 215)
Stir-Fried Spinach with
Sesame Seeds
(page 23)

CTC = 18.5 grams   Calories = 694

Wine: Chardonnay

Peppered Tuna "Tataki"
(page 88)
Tournedos au Poivre with
Balsamic Syrup
(page 121)
Poached Asparagus with
Wasabi Butter
(page 192)
Sautéed Grape Tomatoes
with Shallots (page 218)

CTC = 13.5 grams   Calories = 771

Wine: French Burgundy

Carpaccio of Beef with Mustard Mayonnaise (page 91) Crispy Salmon with Pancetta and Sage (page 181) Slow-Cooked Zucchini with Thyme (page 221) CTC = 4.5 grams Calories = 688 Wine: Pinot Noir or Beaujolais	Broccoli Soup with Basil Butter (page 77) *Bistecca Fiorentina* (page 124) Sautéed Escarole with Garlic (page 201) CTC = 4.5 grams Calories = 580 Wine: Cabernet Sauvignon, any big red from Italy	Baby Spinach Salad with Crispy Bacon (page 101) Veal Loin Chops with Butter and Sage (page 128) Roasted Cauliflower with Cheddar Cheese (page 198) CTC = 5 grams Calories = 631 Wine: Chardonnay or Chianti
Chicken-Pesto Satays (4 skewers each) (page 62) Bay-Steamed Halibut with Lemon Oil (page 171) Oven-Roasted Asparagus with Fried Capers (page 191) CTC = 6 grams Calories = 626 Wine: Sauvignon blanc	Seared Salmon on Lemony Cucumbers (page 97) Asian Chicken with Scallions (page 141) Steamed Broccoli with Stir-Fried Pecans (page 193) CTC = 8.5 grams Calories = 718 Wine: Chenin blanc	Chardonnay Mussels (page 98) Brined Pork Loin with Dry Sherry (page 107) Savoy Cabbage with Bacon and Cumin (page 196) CTC = 10.5 grams Calories = 576 Wine: Sem-Chard from Australia

holiday and special occasion menus

Wine recommendations are made with each menu but are not included in the analyses. To count a glass or two of wine, see page 42.

New Year's Dinner
Little Camembert Popovers (page 59)
Cherrystone Clams with White Balsamic Mignonette (page 84)
Ginger and Chicken Consommé (half portion) (page 72)
Newspaper-Wrapped Fillet of Beef (page 126)
Sautéed Grape Tomatoes with Shallots (page 218)
String Beans with Roasted Garlic Butter (page 205)

CTC = 25 grams Calories = 748

Wine: Brut Champagne/Cabernet Sauvignon

Valentine's Day
Rosettes of Smoked Salmon (page 53)
Fresh Asparagus Soup (page 80)
Sautéed Snapper in Champagne Sauce (page 172)
Sugar Snaps with Yellow Pepper Julienne (page 215)
Chocolate-Dipped Strawberries (page 259)

CTC = 17 grams Calories = 670

Wine: Brut Rose champagne

St. Patrick's Day
Broccoli Soup with Basil Butter (page 77)
St. Patrick's Day Pork and Cabbage (page 110)
Shittake Mushrooms in Sherry-Pepper Cream (page 207)
Red Grapes, Roquefort, and Walnuts (page 235)

CTC = 23 Calories = 719

Beverage: Irish Whiskey or beer

Easter
Chilled Asparagus with Creamy Sesame Dressing (page 93)
Pesto-Crusted Rack of Lamb (page 113)
Sautéed Peas with Pancetta and Mint (page 209)
Roasted Glazed Onions (page 208)

CTC = 25.5 Calories = 714

Wine: Merlot

Mother's Day
Cherry Tomatoes with Herbed Cheese (page 56)
Jade Zucchini Soup with Crab (page 76)
Pesto-Pistachio Chilean Sea Bass (page 166)
String Beans with Roasted Garlic Butter (page 205)

CTC = 15 grams Calories = 583

Wine: Sauvignon Blanc

Father's Day
Chilled Shrimp Cocktail with Low-Carb Cocktail Sauce (page 85)
Bistecca Fiorentina (page 124)
"Creamed" Spinach (page 214)
Roasted Peppers with Balsamic Syrup and Toasted Pine Nuts (page 211)

CTC = 16.5 grams Calories = 672

Wine: Cabernet or Chianti

Fourth of July
Grilled Tuna with Orange-Mint Salsa (page 184)
Smokey Joe Burgers (page 116)
Roasted Glazed Onions (page 208)
Cucumber Salad (page 224) (substitute cilantro, basil, or summery savory for the mint)
Cabbage Slaw (page 225)

CTC = 24 grams Calories = 768

Wine: Chardonnay/Gamay Beaujolais

Newish-Jewish Holiday Dinner

Smoked Salmon "Pâté" with Pita Crisps (page 54)

Garlic Soup with Chicken and Cilantro (page 75)

Golden Capon with 40 Cloves of Garlic (page 153)

Slow-Cooked Zucchini with Thyme (page 221)

Confit of Carrots and Lemon (page 197)

CTC = 22 grams Calories = 776

Wine: Chardonnay or Pinot Noir

Thanksgiving

Cold Oysters with Hot Sausages (page 83)

Madeira-Beef Bouillon (page 73)

Holiday Turkey with Clove-Studded Oranges (page 157)

Roasted Spiced Acorn Squash (page 220)

Sautéed Escarole with Garlic (page 201)

CTC = 22 Calories = 835

Wine: Zinfandel (red) or Shiraz

Christmas Eve

Bombay Shrimp (page 61)

Chardonnay Mussels (page 98)

Pink-and-White "Osso-Buco" (halibut and salmon) (page 182)

Poached Asparagus with Wasabi Butter (page 192)

Wild Rice with Walnut Oil and Scallions (page 227)

CTC = 24 Calories = 804

Wine: Chardonnay/White Burgundy

Christmas Day

Wasabi-Stuffed Shrimp (3 each) (page 55)

Baby Spinach Salad with Crispy Bacon (page 101)

Bay-Smoked Chateaubriand with Truffle-Roasted Salt (page 125)

Brussels Sprouts with Fresh Orange Butter (page 195)

Roasted Portabellos on Rosemary Branches (page 206)

CTC = 13.5 grams Calories = 858

Wine: Cotes du Rhone

Holiday Cocktail Party

Lemon Almonds with Dill (page 49)

Smokey Eggplant-Pesto Dip (page 44)

Whole Wheat Pita Chips (4 each) (page 51)

Roast Beef "Kisses" with Chives (page 58)

Crispy Grape Leaves with Feta Cheese (page 60)

Rosemary Meatballs (page 63)

Prosciutto-Honeydew-Mint Brochettes (page 57)

CTC = 16.5 grams Calories = 478

Wine: Champagne

Holiday Brunch

Prosciutto e Melone (page 90)

Boiled Lobster with Wasabi Mayonnaise (page 86)

Turkish-Style Cucumber Salad (page 223)

Italian Zabaglione (page 254)

CTC = 21.5 grams Calories = 647

Wine: Prosecco (Italian sparkling wine)

the *low carb 1-2-3* food lists

The following four lists indicate the foods that are allowed and or/limited on all low-carb diets. Foods low on the glycemic index (GI) form the basis of healthy low-carb meal plans. Foods higher on the GI should be eaten in moderation or avoided.

the glycemic index

The glycemic index (GI) ranks food by its potential to rapidly increase blood sugar levels. This rise in blood sugar causes surges in insulin levels that have been linked to health problems, including high cholesterol and obesity. The GI is used as a tool for diabetics to help stabilize blood sugar.

Fiber is an integral part of the low-carb equation because it helps us feel full and slows the passage of food through the digestive tract. Because fiber doesn't affect blood sugar levels, we determine our CTCs (Carbs That Count) by subtracting the grams of fiber from total carbohydrates in each recipe. So high-fiber foods are featured prominently on the Foods We Love list on the opposite page.

It's important to keep in mind that eating "good" carbs—the foods on the first two lists—Foods We Love and Foods We Love in Moderation—is essential for our bodies to function. Our brains need good carbohydrates to boost serotonin, the chemical that lifts mood. Our bodies also need carbohydrates to furnish most of the energy we need to live.

Please note that if you are in Phase 1 of the South Beach Diet or in the Induction Phase of Atkins, you should refer to your plan to see what your restrictions are for certain vegetables, fruits, and grains. Remember that these limitations are temporary. After the first 2 weeks, you can freely use every recipe in *Low Carb 1-2-3* as you continue with the next phases of your program.

foods we love

These are the best of the good carbs. These include vegetables and many dairy products. Protein-rich foods such as lean meats, poultry, and fish have negligible carbohydrates and are very low on the GI index.

vegetables

Artichokes	Collards	Okra
Arugula	Cucumber	Onions
Asparagus	Eggplant	Radicchio
Bean sprouts	Endive	Radishes
Bell peppers	Fennel	Snow peas
Bok choy	Jícama	Spinach
Broccoli	Kale	Summer squash
Brussels sprouts	Leeks	String beans
Cabbage	Lettuce	Tomatoes
Cauliflower	Mushrooms	Water chestnuts
Celery	Mustard greens	Watercress
Chayote		

miscellaneous

Cheese and dairy products (low-fat)	Fish (fresh)	Poultry
	Meats (lean)	

foods we love in moderation

These are mostly fruits that should be eaten in smaller portions. Some fruits such as bananas, pineapples, and watermelon should be limited. This list also includes dark chocolate.

fruits

Apples	Grapes	Papaya
Apricots	Honeydew	Peaches
Blackberries	Kiwi	Pears
Blueberries	Lemons	Persimmons
Cantaloupe	Limes	Plums
Carrots	Mandarin oranges	Pomegranates
Cherries	Mango	Strawberries
Figs (fresh)	Nectarines	Tangerines
Grapefruit	Oranges	

miscellaneous

Bulghur wheat

Dark chocolate (70% cocoa)

Legumes (lentils, black beans,
chickpeas, all other beans)

Sweet potatotes/yams

Whole-grain cold cereal
(all-natural, no-sugar-added)

Whole wheat couscous

Wild rice

foods we like but seldom eat

These are high GI foods, which we usually avoid.

fruits and vegetables

Bananas

Beets

Corn

Dried fruit

Parsnips

Pineapple

Raisins

Turnips

Watermelon

miscellaneous

Cornmeal

Fruit juices

Instant hot cereal

Rice- and corn-based cold
cereals

foods we never eat (well, almost never)

These include processed foods that contain partially hydrogenated fats found mainly in packaged
baked goods and snacks, shortenings, and margarine.

Baked beans canned with
added sweeteners

Breads made with white flour,
refined flours, and added
sweeteners (sugar, sucrose,
corn syrup, honey, and
molasses)

Milk chocolate

Nuts with added sugar or

honey, such as honey-
roasted peanuts

Packaged snacks, such as
chips, crackers, granola
bars, trail mix, and power
bars

Pasta and couscous made
with semolina or refined
white flour

Surimi (processed "fish" or
"fake crab" made with
added filler and sugar)

Trans fats (partially
hydrogenated oils)

White flour (enriched or
otherwise)

White rice

Index

Underscored page references indicate boxed text and nutritionist's note.

Conversion Chart

These equivalents have been slightly rounded to make measuring easier.

Volume Measurements

U.S.	Imperial	Metric
¼ tsp	–	1 ml
½ tsp	–	2 ml
1 tsp	–	5 ml
1 Tbsp	–	15 ml
2 Tbsp (1 oz)	1 fl oz	30 ml
¼ cup (2 oz)	2 fl oz	60 ml
⅓ cup (3 oz)	3 fl oz	80 ml
½ cup (4 oz)	4 fl oz	120 ml
⅔ cup (5 oz)	5 fl oz	160 ml
¾ cup (6 oz)	6 fl oz	180 ml
1 cup (8 oz)	8 fl oz	240 ml

Weight Measurements

U.S.	Metric
1 oz	30 g
2 oz	60 g
4 oz (¼ lb)	115 g
5 oz (⅓ lb)	145 g
6 oz	170 g
7 oz	200 g
8 oz (½ lb)	230 g
10 oz	285 g
12 oz (¾ lb)	340 g
14 oz	400 g
16 oz (1 lb)	455 g
2.2 lb	1 kg

Length Measurements

U.S.	Metric
¼"	0.6 cm
½"	1.25 cm
1"	2.5 cm
2"	5 cm
4"	11 cm
6"	15 cm
8"	20 cm
10"	25 cm
12" (1')	30 cm

Pan Sizes

U.S.	Metric
8" cake pan	20 × 4 cm sandwich or cake tin
9" cake pan	23 × 3.5 cm sandwich or cake tin
11" × 7" baking pan	28 × 18 cm baking tin
13" × 9" baking pan	32.5 × 23 cm baking tin
15" × 10" baking pan	38 × 25.5 cm baking tin (Swiss roll tin)
1½ qt baking dish	1.5 liter baking dish
2 qt baking dish	2 liter baking dish
2 qt rectangular baking dish	30 × 19 cm baking dish
9" pie plate	22 × 4 or 23 × 4 cm pie plate
7" or 8" springform pan	18 or 20 cm springform or loose-bottom cake tin
9" × 5" loaf pan	23 × 13 cm or 2 lb narrow loaf tin or pâté tin

Temperatures

Fahrenheit	Centigrade	Gas
140°	60°	–
160°	70°	–
180°	80°	–
225°	105°	¼
250°	120°	½
275°	135°	1
300°	150°	2
325°	160°	3
350°	180°	4
375°	190°	5
400°	200°	6
425°	220°	7
450°	230°	8
475°	245°	9
500°	260°	–